The Complete
Allergy Relief Handbook
STOP ITCHING, SNEEZING, WHEEZING, AND COUGHING

by Randall Earl Dunford

Magni Group, Inc.

ISBN: 1-882330-86-2

Manufactured in the United States of America

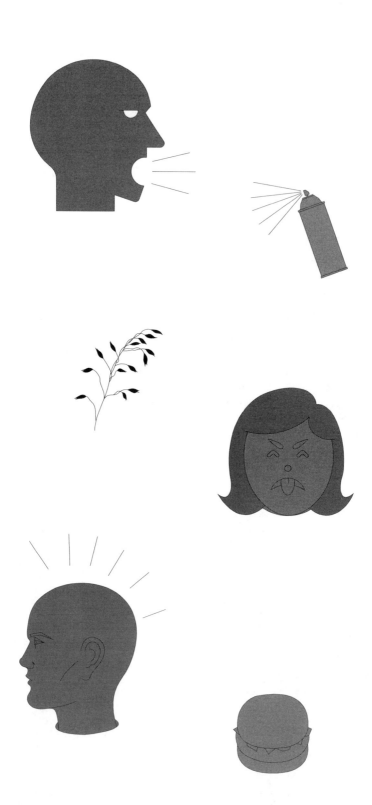

Contents

Part 3: Solutions

Part 1:
Introduction

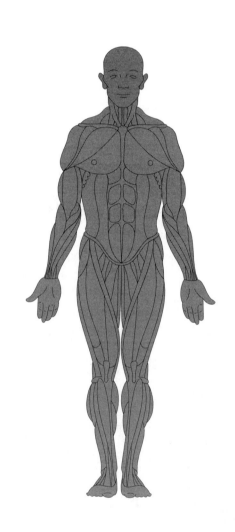

Chapter 1
The Facts about Allergy

What is an allergy? Obviously, this question must be answered before one holds any chance of determining if he or she is suffering from this uncomfortable, sometimes serious, occasionally deadly dysfunction, or battling an illness of another nature.

Some confine their interpretation of an allergy to nothing more than an attack of hay fever (allergic rhinitis), sometimes called pollinosis. At best, most regard allergies as any number of annoying respiratory difficulties brought on by the inhalation of airborne substances such as dust, pollen or mold. The problem, unfortunately, takes on a much broader scope than that.

In reality, an allergy (from the Greek words *allos* and *ergon*, meaning "other action") is an adverse reaction in a person who has previously been exposed to a foreign substance (known as an antigen) and is exposed to it again. In the initial encounter, the body produces proteins (called antibodies) that are tailor-made to match specific substances in order to fight off infections and disease. This first exposure creates no apparent problem but sometimes something goes awry and the body becomes sensitized to the substance. The next time the body is exposed to that same substance, normally harmless (or a normally tolerable dose of a potentially harmful substance), its immune system mistakenly regards that substance as a threat and releases histamine and similar natural chemicals. Normal amounts of these chemicals are harmless, but higher concentrations, as are produced in this case, will generate the problems that cause unwanted symptoms.

To make matters worse, your body continues to produce these chemicals even when you have removed yourself from contact with the allergen, perpetuating if not intensifying the symptoms.

These symptoms can take many forms and the list of substances that can be involved is not by any means short. The middle-age executive who suffers with watery eyes and a runny nose may have developed an allergy to pollen. The elderly gentleman who is plagued with stomach aches might be allergic to eggs. Animal dander

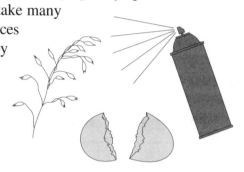

There are many substances capable of triggering allergic symptoms.

could be the cause of a little girl's asthma. Or a cleaning solution might just be producing a homemaker's skin rash.

Table 1

Substances that can Cause Allergies	
Animal dander	Insect venom
Chemicals (household and industrial)	Medication
Dust	Mold
Dust mites	Pesticides
Food and beverages	Pollen

An allergy can even masquerade as another illness such as arthritis, heart disease, colitis, vaginitis, gallbladder dysfunction and many others, or it can complicate these very maladies. Furthermore, allergies sometimes get the blame for learning disabilities, autism, alcoholism, irritability, anxiety, depression, hyperactivity, bed-wetting and criminal behavior.

In addition, allergies sometimes begot other allergies in an individual. For instance, one may have developed a sensitivity to pollen and later fall victim to mold spores. Or one who has become susceptible to corn may develop an equal sensitivity to other grains such as rice.

Also, one allergy can aggravate another, sometimes of an entirely different nature. This can be observed when one who is allergic to both eggs and vehicle exhaust emissions reacts more severely while in heavy traffic only after eating eggs.

An allergic reaction can begin immediately or be delayed for a day or more. In some cases, an allergy may not surface until later in life. It can be of only minor annoyance or become more serious. In the worst case scenario, one can be attacked by what is known as anaphylactic shock (anaphylaxis), a potentially fatal condition characterized by a rapid pulse, falling blood pressure, swollen throat, and fluid in the lungs.

Some individuals suffer with an allergy only at certain times. This is known as a seasonal allergy. A good example is hay fever, which typically makes its presence felt only during pollen season. The more unfortunate suffer from what is called a perennial allergy; that is, they are in a constant state of distress, such as that induced from automobile exhaust. There are others more unfortunate still who are stricken with both.

Allergies can affect young and old, professionals and laymen, men and women. They have no respect for ethnic groups nor do they recognize any geographic bounds.

Unfortunately, drug treatments are not always effective because skin tests are not conclusive in every case. In fact, one can even develop an allergy to the medication itself.

Estimates are that half of the world's population is beset by allergies. Some experts believe as many as 60% of those seeking medical help, young and old alike, may possess symptoms that are either caused or complicated by allergies.

Table 2

Kinds of Physical Disorders Sometimes Mimicked or Aggravated by Allergies

Arthritis	Headaches (especially migraine)
Asthma	Hearing difficulties
Bed-wetting	Kidney disorder
Colitis	Menopause problems
Epileptic seizures	Ulcers
Gallbladder dysfunction	Vaginitis
Heart disease	

Table 3

Kinds of Mental Disorders Sometimes Caused by Allergies

Alcoholism	Criminal behavior
Anxiety	Depression
Autism	Hyperactivity
Compulsive eating	Irritability

What Kind of Allergy Do You Have?

There are four basic scenarios for allergies. Allergens can be breathed (airborne substances), ingested (food, drink or medication), injected (medication) or by direct contact of the skin surface (chemicals, clothing, plants, etc.). The latter usually manifests itself into usually either a respiratory allergy, a digestive allergy or a skin allergy.

If the respiratory tract is affected, one will likely suffer with a runny nose, watery eyes, sneezing and the like. Should the digestive system be struck, the symptoms may come in the form of nausea, vomiting or diarrhea. If the skin becomes irritated, hives or blisters may surface.

Any internal part of the body, however, can be afflicted. This includes the less obvious such as muscles, joints, and the brain, as well as the other internal organs. That's because anything inhaled is absorbed by the blood-vessel-rich alveoli walls of the lungs, diffused into the bloodstream, and carried by the red blood cells to every part of the body. In addition, contaminants can enter the digestive system from swallowed particle-laden sputum that one fails to eliminate when coughing or sneezing. In similar fashion, ingestants ultimately find their way to the rest of the body and can produce symptoms in the respiratory passages or on the skin, simulating an airborne or skin allergy.

The Many Symptoms Produced by Allergies

With all of this, it's no wonder the symptoms of allergy are wide and varied. Well-recognized symptoms include runny or stuffy nose, sneezing, coughing, watery or itchy eyes, wheezing, and hives or other skin irritations. Lesser known symptoms consist of headaches, tinnitus, nausea, vomiting, diarrhea, constipation, muscle aches, join pain, irregular heartbeats, cold hands and feet, vertigo, and fatigue. Refer to table 4 for a more comprehensive list of symptoms.

Table 4

Symptoms That can be Produced by Allergy

Cold hands and feet	Itchy eyes	Stuffy nose
Constipation	Itchy skin	Swollen eyes
Coughing	Join pain	Tinnitus
Diarrhea	Muscle aches	Vertigo
Dry skin	Nausea	Vomiting
Fatigue	Red spots on skin	Watery eyes
Headaches	Runny nose	Wheezing
Hives	Sneezing	
Irregular heartbeats	Stomach ache	

Hopefully by now, you have a better conception of just what an allergy is and what to expect of it. If you or your doctor have not yet identified your allergy, you may have isolated the problem by now or have even uncovered a hidden allergy within yourself or someone you love. At any rate, the previous information has probably given you some serious food for thought. But it is most likely too general to offer enough help, so before attempting to nail down the solutions, let's build a greater understanding of the matter by taking a look at the agents that can, and all too often do, trigger allergies.

Part 2:
Identifying the Allergens

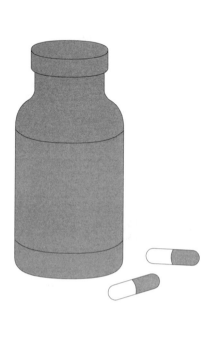

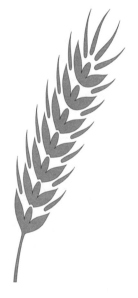
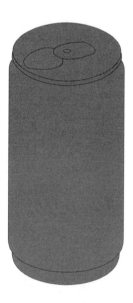

Chapter 2
Airborne Enemies

Of the many substances capable of triggering an allergic response, the most widely recognized is probably particulate airborne matter such as dust, pollen and mold. There are other substances riding the air as well, which can also prove damaging to the human system, in the form of gases that our industrial existence has brought about. Let's discuss the particulate matter first.

Dust

Dust catches the blame for many allergies. We are forced to live with this grayish, powdery material on a constant basis, always inhaling it to some extent. We have no other choice unless we shift our existence to outer space.

But this substance is really not as bad as it is cracked up to be. Few people develop an allergy to dust. The problem usually lies not with the dust itself, but with the particles that hitchhike on the dust. There is an incredible and diverse collection of matter that is conveyed through the air via dust. Dust mites, mold spores, pollen, dander, pesticide powders, insect fragments, insect excretions, paint chips, bits of plaster, wallpaper flakes, bits of cotton and wool, residue from cosmetics, fireplace soot, and even food remnants are just a few examples. Refer to Table 5 for a more comprehensive list.

If you *do* have an allergy to dust, you undoubtedly suffer from sinusitis or another respiratory condition. Inside houses and buildings, symptoms may be initiated or made worse whenever portable fans are put in use, or when air conditioning or heating is first turned on at the beginning of a new season, because of an accumulation of particles around the vents and places in direct contact with the blowing air. Added to this is the dust that escapes the air filter. Heating systems are worse because warmer air possesses a greater capacity for holding particles.

Unknown to most, the introduction of heat can make matters worse in another way, if not cause the problem in the first place. The high operating temperature of the elements of an electric heater or the heat produced from burning incandescent light bulbs is capable of chemically altering dust. This has been dubbed as "fried dust" by the late renown allergist Theron Randolph.

Heated or not, the hustle and bustle of daily activity keeps a lot of dust particles aloft. The larger ones tend to settle first, but the smaller, more easily breathable, remain suspended longer—and are more readily disturbed—because of their lighter weight.

If you think you have a dust allergy, consider the other particles that could be flying about, whether as part of the dust itself or moving separately in the air.

Table 5

Particles that can be Conveyed Through the Air via Dust	
Algae	Insect fragments
Animal dander	Mold spores
Cellulose shreds	Paint chips
Cosmetics residue	Pesticide powders
Cotton fibers	Plaster bits
Detergents	Pollen grains
Dust mites	Wallpaper flakes
Fireplace soot	Wood particles
Food remnants	Wool fibers
Insect excretions	

Dust Mites

Dust mites (dermatophagoides), whose existence were unknown until the 1960s, are more likely to be the cause of an allergy than that of dust; and truly they are a common component. One study group of entomologists collected dust from 64 homes in the eastern part of the United States and found dust mites inhabiting nearly two-thirds of the samples. And this was only one test. Some estimates put that percentage at 99%.

These microscopic arthropods, which live in temperatures above 50° Fahrenheit, feed on flakes of skin we regularly shed, drawing nourishment from keratin, the protein that it contains. They also dine on food particles. Dust mites are especially fond of humid conditions. They also like darkness—and the warmer the temperature, the better. They multiply fiercely, each female laying as many as 50 eggs and producing a new generation every 3 weeks. You won't stand a chance of spotting them with the naked eye, but chances are they are present around you, outdoors as well as in. Some of their favorite breeding grounds inside are upholstery and bedding in damp rooms. (Sweating and bed-wetting contribute to this.) A double bed alone may furnish a home for not much less than 2 million dust mites. Carpeting and curtains are other areas where they can be found. When they feel the suction of a vacuum cleaner, they have an uncanny way of clinging to the surface they are occupying.

They have been known to cause severe itch, and not only can one develop an allergy to dust mites, but also from their excrements! According to David Rousseau, author of *Your Home, Your Health, and Well-Being*, "Their presence is the major reason why dust causes reactions among allergy sufferers, even when pollen and house pets are not present."

Other symptoms that can be associated with dust mite allergy are rhinitis, asthma and eczema. Diarrhea, vomiting, stomach cramps may also result along with the production of nasal polyps. When dust mite allergy causes rhinitis in children, it can be accompanied by what is called "glue ear," a condition that results from an excessive accumulation of mucus in the nasal passages that works its way up into the eustachian tube to create an obstruction.

And it may seem contradictory, but although dust mites flourish during summer months, those affected may actually find their symptoms worse in winter. This is because by the winter season these tiny creatures have died, and their dried up bodies have broken down into fragments. These fragments, being obviously smaller than the full-sized mite, can more easily pass through heater filters, remain aloft longer and more easily reach the respiratory tract.

Mold

Molds are microscopic organisms necessary to life that fall under the biological heading of fungi. They reproduce via tiny seedlike spores, which are released from colonies and lifted into the air and can be found everywhere throughout the world. Of the many hundreds of species, some are used beneficially, as in food processing for flavoring soft drinks, alcoholic beverages, cheeses, confections and other foodstuffs; in the manufacture of drugs such as penicillin and streptomycin; and in making silver plating possible. This suggests that mold may be at the root of the problem for some of those who think they have an allergy to certain foods or drugs.

Out-of-doors, the mold season generally extends from late spring to fall, except in the southern regions of the United States, where it can be a year-round affair. Undisturbed accumulations in spots least exposed to sunlight, such as on tree bark, logs, leaves, soil, and the like can be a thing of beauty, often blooming into a number of intriguing shapes and colors. Mold is also capable of growing on a number of other objects, including grasses, straw, and hay, in addition to crops such as wheat and oats. An adverse reaction, therefore, to some of these items could be a mold allergy in disguise.

There is no doubt that mold can be a problem for individuals when spending time outside, but it posses an even greater threat inside. Not only does some of it find its way inside, but some kinds of mold proliferate inside as well as out and become what is often termed "mildew." It is estimated that as many as 20 million Americans may have become susceptible to even minute doses.

Like dust mites, molds breed in damp areas. Buildings erected over swamp lands or other such wet areas can harbor mold permanently unless corrected by construction. Also, houses in wooded areas can be particularly vulnerable. And ground-floor apartments and first-floor offices are often more humid and therefore more conducive to mold growth than upper levels.

Inside, kitchens and bathrooms are by far the most likely to harbor mold. Leaky plumbing and sluggish drains make matters all the worse. Basements can also give mold a home as can attics under a leaky roof, not to mention improperly maintained air ducts, and for that matter any room with moist walls. But mold can multiply anywhere indoors as it is also dependent on darkness and the absence of ventilation for survival. A lot of household items also offer breeding grounds for mold. These include damp towels, clothes and blankets; foam rubber pillows; leather goods; mattresses; shoes; stuffed furniture; vaporizers; humidifiers; carpeting; aquariums; books and magazines; and pet litter. Refer to table 6 for a more comprehensive list.

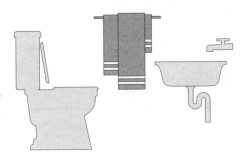

Due to the high volume of moisture present, bathrooms are one of the most likely areas to harbor mold.

What can be seen that has accumulated, however, will not affect anyone. It's what ultimately dries out and detaches itself from the accumulation that gets into the air for a possible entry into the respiratory tract that matters. But as long as it is allowed to keep growing, an ample supply will exist to make life miserable for some.

Common symptoms of a mold allergy are a stuffy nose, runny eyes, mental confusion, asthma, depression, and fatigue. Susceptibility to mold can even masquerade as multiple sclerosis, which includes such symptoms as numbness and weakness of the limbs. Some MS patients, in fact, have achieved partial relief from their disease by eliminating airborne contaminants such as mold from their surroundings. The same also applies to other central nervous system disorders such as cerebral palsy and polio.

Table 6

Favorite Breeding Grounds for Dust Mites and Mold	
Air ducts	Leaky plumbing
Aquariums	Leather goods
Blankets	Magazines
Books	Mattresses
Carpeting	Pet litter
Clothes	Shoes
Curtains	Stuffed furniture
Damp towels	Towels
Foam rubber pillows	Upholstery
Humidifiers	Vaporizers

Pollen

Anyone who has picked up a dandelion has undoubtedly noticed the yellow "powder" that so liberally comes off on the hands. This, of course, is pollen—the fertilizing element that is responsible for perpetuating plant reproduction. Near the surface of each pollen grain are enzymes. These enzymes, which are proteins, are the actual allergens, ordinarily released from the grain to help it enter the stigma of a receptive flower.

Some plants are self-pollinating. Usually, however, pollen is transferred by insects, birds or the wind. In rare cases it is even transferred by water. Some species, such as goldenrod, are pollinated by both insects and wind. There are many kinds of pollen, each produced from its particular species, including those of grasses, trees and weeds.

Unfortunately, pollen plays one of the largest roles as an instigator of respiratory ailments. According to American Academy of Allergy estimates, 35 million Americans are troubled by pollen. It is, in fact, the most common adult allergen. The usual reaction is hay fever. Other problems that have been known to occur are asthma and depression.

In fact, a surprising number of chronic hay fever sufferers eventually develop asthma. An individual may only be affected by a specific kind of pollen, but once he or she has contracted an allergy to it, it's possible to later develop a sensitivity to other kinds as well. Also, it is not uncommon for those who are sensitive to mold to be equally affected by pollen, nor is it unusual for persons to react differently to different kinds of pollen. In fact, just one microspore can trouble a highly-sensitive individual.

How Pollen Produces Allergic Symptoms

A pollen grain is designed to penetrate the stigma of a compatible flower in order to reach the female egg cell nestled deeply inside, where it is to deposit a male cell. In order to do so, the pollen grain must rapidly release chemicals that help the plant determine if it is a matching species and, if so, discharge more chemicals (in the form of enzymes) to help it eat its way into the stigma of the prospective flower. What triggers this response is moisture contained within the stigma. But if a pollen grain should enter the nose while in dutiful search of a mate, this same chemical barrage is evoked by the moisture in the nasal passage. Effects are not always immediate. It may require 2 seasons, or as many as 5, before allergy symptoms surface.

The pollen season can be miserably long in warmer climates where the growing period is of a lengthier duration. Moreover, those susceptible to more than one kind of pollen must face an even greater burden. With few exceptions, trees make the largest contribution in springtime, grass presents the heaviest load during early summer, and weeds are the major culprit by fall. Virtually all plant life is capable of generating pollen until it has gone to seed.

Weeds are the worst offenders—particularly ragweed, because it is so prolific. One of its favorite habitats is freshly disturbed ground (a special invitation being uprooted dirt at construction sites), but it grows abundantly in any soil. It is such a hearty breed that ragweed seeds have been known to germinate 40 years after production. Although relatively inconspicuous, it can be recognized by its coarse, hairy stems, divided leaves (with 3 to 5-inch lobes), and long spikes of tiny greenish-yellow flowers. There are hundreds of varieties. Allergists in the U. S. estimate that in excess of 250,000 tons of ragweed pollen are picked up by the atmosphere annually, and it has been detected as high into the atmosphere as 2 miles up and as far as 400 miles out to sea. A single plant is capable of producing as many as one trillion pollen grains! The American College of Allergy, Asthma, and Immunology estimates that 75% of all hay fever victims are allergic to ragweed pollen.

Grasses are the second worst offenders—and there are more cross-reactions among them than that of the other plant families. Of the some 4,000 species, Bermuda grass contains the most allergenic pollen. In the mid-south and Gulf states, it is a usual part of the landscape. Timothy grass, meanwhile, poses a problem in Great Britain. Other particularly potential culprits include Johnson grass, Kentucky bluegrass, orchard grass, redtop grass and sweet vernal grass. Even oats and wheat, which fall under the category of grasses, can spell trouble for some after they have been cultivated.

Some examples of the kind of trees that generate allergenic pollen are ash, oak, elm, box elder, hickory, mountain cedar and birch. Elms are more prevalent in the northern United States, while cedars are common in the West and in south Texas, and birch can be found more notably in the northern portion of the country. Some kinds, such as oaks, exist in every state except Alaska and Hawaii.

Trees, grass and weed pollen are all readily carried aloft (sometimes thousands of miles) because of their smaller size and the fact that these

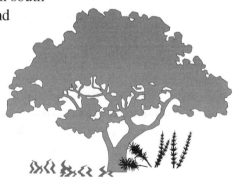

Weeds are the most troublesome culprits in regard to pollen allergies, followed by grasses and then trees.

pollens are not particularly sticky. There is nothing to prevent it from landing on flowers, either, so take heed if roses, iris or the like are part of your life—especially if bringing them indoors.

As a general rule, flower pollen (*i. e.*, that produced from ornamental flowering plants such as roses, as opposed to that of plants considered less desirable, such as ragweed) is not as likely to trigger allergies because, not only is a smaller quantity of it produced, it is larger and heavier, and excessively sticky, and therefore not as easily transported by the wind. Its transfer is usually dependent upon insects and birds, which are attracted by the colorful petals and sweet fragrances of the flowers that produce it.

And take note of this fact. House plans rarely produce pollen. It's the mold that grows on their leaves and soil surfaces that pose potential allergy problems.

Pollen is at its worst on hot, dry, windy days, and less troublesome when it is cool, cloudy and windless. Conditions are also more favorable when it rains because water washes it out of the atmosphere, and when humidity is high because pollen is not released then. Levels are generally highest in late evening and early morning, so keep this in mind when airing out the house or going for a walk.

Many hay fever sufferers, however, have avoided outdoor activity during pollen season, only to find little or no relief. The truth is that pollen can, and often does, make its way into the house and other buildings. Not unlike other particulate matter, pollen can be brought indoors on hair, clothing, shoes, pets, insects and rodents. Although pollen grains, in their original state, are big enough to be stopped by conventional heating and air conditioning filters, they can easily break down into fragments small enough to slip through not only those filters but inexpensive air purifiers advertised as possessing the capability of screening particles smaller than the smallest pollen size. In the winter season, any pollen that is still trapped inside one's living quarters will linger and continue to produce symptoms in a sensitive individual who then mistakenly draws the conclusion that the problem is not from pollen.

Hay fever, of course, is the usual response in those who have become sensitive to pollen. It often starts with an itchy sensation in the nose, mouth, throat and eyes and graduates to sneezing and a runny or stuffy nose. Hay fever, however, is not the only consequence of a pollen allergy. Sometimes digestive problems, such as an upset stomach, or even colitis can result presumably because of the ingestion of food on which pollen has settled or because of pollen that has been inhaled and swallowed. Skin reactions such as hives or eczema can also surface from either direct contact or via the bloodstream, which the pollen has invaded through the blood vessels in the nose.

Outdoor Gaseous Pollutants

Particulate matter is not the only problem for allergy sufferers by far. Our industrial existence has brought about countless other pollutants, many of gaseous natures. The chief problem with these substances is that they exist on a molecular level and conventional air filters or filter masks offer no defense against them.

Metropolitan areas are home to petroleum refineries, smelting plants, paint manufacturers, plastic factories, coal-fired electric power plants, refuse incinerators, fireplace smoke, and the like. Also not to be overlooked are emissions from the exhaust of motor vehicles whether it be automobiles, trucks or buses. If the engines are in disrepair, all the worse. And fumes from jet aircraft add significantly to this as well. In fact, the emissions from one jet upon takeoff is equivalent to that produced by as many as 7,000 passing cars! Diesel fuel discharges are an even greater threat than those of standard gasoline engines because it is composed of heavier chemicals and it vaporizes at a much higher temperature.

Vehicle Exhaust Emissions and Hay Fever

Exposure to an inordinate amount of vehicle exhaust fumes appears to encourage hay fever brought on by pollen. A Japanese study that compared people from different areas showed that those with the highest incidence of hay fever were living along busy streets lined with red cedar trees and, in fact, were 3 times more likely to be stricken than those dwelling near forests of red cedar well away from the beaten track.

Released into the air as a result of all this are a multitude of chemicals. The ones of primary concern consist of carbon monoxide, sulfur oxides, nitrogen oxides and hydrocarbons—but any of them can pose a threat. What's worse, these vapors and gases carry with them particulate matter as well. When the gaseous and particulate matter combines with moisture, smog is created.

Some five hundred million pounds of chemicals are produced annually. The number of compounds in common use in the U. S. today is estimated at over 60,000, and that figure is growing steadily. It is said that on the average, one new compound is synthesized every minute!

One may seek refuge from these outdoor pollutants by spending more time inside. This may help, but often doses of these chemicals make their way in, where they become trapped and circulate through the air system. One may also consider it safer to be inside a car rather than around its exhaust, but unknown to many, the gases—as well as other pollutants—can be pulled into the vehicle via windows and air vents.

If these airborne substances were all that triggered allergies it would be bad enough. But there is more, much more. Next let's take a look at how food can affect the human system in an allergic sense.

Chapter 3
The Truth about Food (and Beverages)

The pastime of eating is typically an enjoyable experience and most all of us look forward to our meals. Unfortunately, foods can trigger allergy. This also includes most beverages, as they are derived from food substances. Food allergy is not uncommon. Estimates are that well over half the world's population is affected. About 1 out of every 20, in fact, are so sensitive to certain foods that even a morsel of one of the offending edibles can spark an immediate reaction.

Physicians admit that skin tests for food allergies are less reliable than those for inhalant allergies, thus food allergies can be a lot harder to isolate. Besides that, symptoms don't always manifest themselves into digestive problems. This is further complicated by the fact that most heavily processed foods contain a large number of other ingredients. Add to this the fact that reactions may be delayed until after the next meal is consumed, or even longer.

On occasion, allergic effects can be immediate. One, for instance, can experience itching or swelling in the mouth just after consumption of the troublesome food. Usually, however, symptoms are delayed until the food is processed by the digestive system. At that point, distress may erupt in the form of nausea or diarrhea. As the food allergen makes its way to the remainder of the body, symptoms can become more varied, such as those of joint pain or skin rashes. This may require a few hours or be put off for a day or more.

If one suspects an allergy of this nature, he or she can be fooled into blaming the wrong food. One could have developed a sensitivity to fish eaten the evening before, but mistakenly comes to believe it is because of the eggs consumed for breakfast the next morning.

To complicate the issue still further, one may tolerate a food on some occasions, but not others. That doesn't necessarily mean you don't have an allergy to it. In this case, it could be that the body is responding to an accumulative effect. A certain quantity of the food can be tolerated, but over time the body finally says it has had enough and rebels. This can also take place in another way. One might be allergic to several foods, either of which he or she might be able to tolerate alone. But if eaten in combination it becomes enough to put the body's defenses over the edge. This especially applies to foods that are closely related, such as tomato and potato. And in another variation of this scenario, certain foods may give one trouble only after he or she has been exposed to an unusually large quantity of an airborne allergen such as mold.

The kinds of food that most commonly cause allergies are:

• corn
• eggs
• milk
• wheat
• nuts
• fish

Other foods that quite often, but less likely to trigger allergies include chocolate, pork and yeast. On the list of those that sometimes induce allergic responses are cheese, beef, chicken, mushrooms, bananas and melons. Some foods less frequently cause a problem, such as apples, barley, beets, oats, salmon, carrots, lettuce, honey, squash, apricots, rice, peaches, pineapples and rye.

Let's examine some of the most likely culprits in more detail.

Corn

When one thinks of this grain, he or she usually pictures corn on the cob or a can of corn. If an allergy is involved, avoiding the real thing, it is reasoned, will solve the problem. But not so.

Those with a sensitivity to corn may find it particularly challenging to remove all traces of this food from their diet because there are so many processed foods that contain corn sugar or corn syrup (often declared on the label as "dextrose" or "high fructose corn syrup" among numerous others). Among the most notable are bacon; ham; sausage; cakes; breads; pastries; doughnuts; pancake mixes; biscuits; pie crusts and cream pies; cereals; cheeses; cookies; candy; ice cream; jams, jellies and preserves; powdered sugar; ketchup and sauces used for meats; vegetables and sundaes; salad dressings; sandwich spreads; soups; syrups; baking powders; distilled vinegar; and canned fruit and vegetables.

In addition, there are a number of beverages included in this category; namely, instant coffee and tea, fruit juices, sweetened condensed milk, soft drinks, beer, ale, whiskey, gin and some soybean milks. Refer to table 7 for a more comprehensive list of foods and beverages that commonly contain corn derivatives.

Add to this an unsuspected item in the form of plastic food wrappers, whose inner surface is sometimes coated with cornstarch as well as a few seemingly unrelated products: aspirin (and other medications in tablet form), cough syrups, chewing gum and some brands of toothpaste.

It's easy to see, then, how one can attempt to halt allergic symptoms by consuming an apparently cornless meal that consists of cured ham, a can of English peas, french fries with ketchup, a biscuit, a slice of coconut cream pie and a soft drink, yet be ingesting corn with every swallow.

Common reactions from corn include stuffy nose, sneezing and intestinal distress, in addition to hives.

Table 7

Processed Foods and Beverages that Commonly Contain Corn Derivatives

Ale	Margarine
Bacon	Pancake mixes
Baking powder	Pancake syrup
Barbecue sauce	Pastries
Beer	Pickles (sweet)
Biscuits	Pie crusts
Breads	Pies (cream)
Cakes	Preserves
Candy	Pudding
Cereals	Relish
Cheeses	Salad dressings
Coffee (instant)	Salt (iodized)
Cookies	Sandwich spreads
Corn chips	Sausage
Doughnuts	Soft drinks
Flour (bleached wheat)	Soups
Fruit (canned)	Soybean milk
Fruit juices	Spaghetti sauce
Gin	Sugar (powdered)
Grits	Sweetened condensed milk
Ham	Syrups
Hominy	Tea (instant)
Ice cream	Vanilla flavoring
Jams	Vegetables (canned and frozen)
Jellies	Vinegar (distilled)
Ketchup and other sauces	Whiskey
Malt and malt syrup	Yogurt

Eggs

Recognized as a good source of protein, this commodity is common at the breakfast table. But eggs contain exceptionally large concentrations of cholesterol and one would do well to limit the quantity consumed.

Those with an allergy to eggs, however, find themselves forced to eliminate them from their diet. If all that was necessary was to give up the "sunny-side ups," life would be simple enough. But like corn, eggs are a constituent of a lot of other foods. They turn up in cakes, pies, pancakes, waffles, puddings, ice cream, marshmallows, salad dressing (particularly Caesar), stuffing for seafood dishes, and are the basic ingredient of mayonnaise, as well as custards and noodles—and, of course, eggnog. They can also be included in potato salad, milkshakes and meat balls. Wine and malted cocoa drinks are also on this list. In addition, eggs are often used to create milk or foam toppings on specialty coffee drinks. One can also have a problem with eggs if taking a vaccine that has been grown on egg cultures!

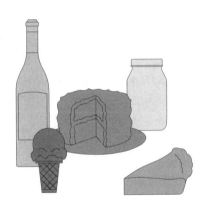

Eggs can be found not only in cakes, ice cream and pies but in a number of other processed foods, including wine.

Interestingly, one may possess a sensitivity to only part of the egg. Either the yolk or the white can be the culprit, but the white portion usually proves to be the allergen because most of the proteins that are capable of triggering allergic reactions exist there. Additionally, one may be able to tolerate eggs only if cooked more completely. A hard-boiled egg may be acceptable, for instance, but not the fried variety, especially because, in this case, the yellow remains virtually uncooked. Occasionally, a person develops such a sensitivity that even the consumption of chicken becomes a problem. This, however, may be because eggs sometimes contain measures of the hen's blood. Also, those with an allergy to chicken eggs will likely be allergic to those of other species, such as turkey or duck.

Table 8

Processed Foods that Commonly Contain Eggs

Cakes	Oatmeal
Custards	Pancakes
Ice cream	Pies
Malted cocoa drinks	Potato salad
Marshmallows	Puddings
Mayonnaise	Salad dressing
Meat balls	Stuffing for seafood dishes
Milkshakes	Tartar sauce
Muffins	Waffles
Noodles	Wine

Milk

The ever popular cow's milk has long been touted as an excellent food. While it's high in protein, it has been responsible for a huge number of allergies—especially in children, undoubedly because children are encouraged to drink it. In fact, allergists rank milk as the number one cause of food allergy.

As in the case of corn and eggs, milk or one of its derivatives can be concealed in other foods. A milk allergy sufferer may find trouble in gravies, cream, cheese (including some soy cheeses), yogurt, ice cream, certain breads, some margarines, cakes and other baked goods, soups, creamed vegetables (including mashed potatoes), chocolate and puddings and other desserts. And believe it or not, creamers and cheese marked as "nondiary" are also on this list!

Allergic problems can stem from one or more of three components of milk: fat, proteins or carbohydrates (sugars).

Many have developed a problem with lactose, the principle carbohydrate. Most physicians regard this as lactose intolerance rather than an allergy because of a deficiency of lactase (an enzyme designed specifically to digest lactose), which is secreted by villi (hairlike protrusions along the intestinal wall). Some, however, hold the consensus that this problem develops *as the result* of an allergy because food allergy usually causes intestinal inflammation that damages the villi. As one of the functions of the villi is to absorb fat, this suggests one reason why a person may also develop adverse reactions to the fat in milk.

The milk protein known as casein can also be a culprit. Heating milk breaks down this protein as well as some of the other 25 that exist there, making it possible for a number of individuals to tolerate this food, yet others are only able to get away with drinking raw milk.

Other products can become adulterated with milk from food outlets that use the same utensils for slicing unrelated items such as celery and cheese. The same scenario holds true when packaging or manufacturing equipment is employed for different products.

Approximately 25% of those plagued with airborne allergies also react to milk. Common symptoms of milk allergy are runny nose, congestion, wheezing, stomach ache, bloating, vomiting and bloody diarrhea. Milk allergy can also cause rashes and even ear infections.

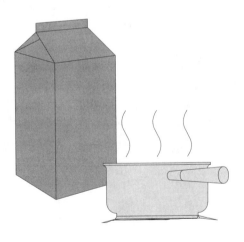

Heating milk breaks down much of its protein, allowing some allergic individuals to tolerate it.

Table 9

Processed Foods that may or do Contain Milk or Milk Derivatives

Breads
Butter
Cakes (and other baked goods)
Cheeses (including soy cheeses)
Chocolate
Cookies
Crackers
Cream (including nondairy)
Creamed vegetables (including mashed potatoes)
Custard
Gravies
Ice cream
Margarine
Nuts (coated)
Pancakes
Pasta sauce
Puddings (and other desserts)
Salad dressing
Soups
Teas (flavored)
Whipped toppings
Yogurt

Wheat

Who is not familiar with the Biblical quote, "Man shall not live by bread alone?" There are many who find they must not live by it at all. This staple is usually a part of just about every meal and its almost always made from wheat. It is the major source of wheat in our diet.

Actually, it's a protein called gluten that the wheat contains that's a chief cause of many allergies. It's presence in wheat is what gives breads and other baked goods a light spongy texture due to its elastic nature. Gluten is also found in other grains such as oats and rye, but to a lesser degree. That means some may be able to tolerate these other grains, but not wheat. Unfortunately, some are so sensitive to gluten that they are unable to consume any of these grains. It is also possible one could have an allergy to the yeast used to turn the dough into bread rather than wheat and not be the wiser. So if one removes all wheat from his or her diet and still experiences allergic symptoms, chances are an allergy to gluten or yeast exists rather than to the wheat itself.

Wheat is no different than corn, eggs or milk when it comes to hiding in other foods. Some items which include or could include wheat or wheat gluten are luncheon meats, frankfurters, sausage, cheese spreads with cereal fillers, canned or frozen foods with thick sauces (including soups), gravies, dumplings, cakes, crackers, biscuits, pancakes, waffles, pretzels, casseroles, ice cream, candy and baking powder. And, of course, don't overlook cereal. In addition, some kinds of chewing gum earn a spot on this list. Refer to table 10 for a more comprehensive listing.

Likely symptoms in those with a wheat allergy are digestive difficulties such as cramps, indigestion, gas, diarrhea and bloating. Other common, seemingly unrelated symptoms, can also surface in the form of eczema as well as asthma and other respiratory problems.

Table 10

Processed Foods that May or Do Contain Wheat

Baking powder
Biscuits
Cakes
Candy
Canned or frozen foods (with thick sauces)
Casseroles
Cereal
Cheese spreads (with cereal fillers)
Crackers
Doughnuts
Dumplings
Fish patties
Frankfurters
Gravies
Ice cream
Luncheon meats
Meat loaf
Meat patties
Noodles
Pancakes
Pasta
Pastries
Pies
Pretzels
Sausage
Soups
Waffles
White vinegar

Nuts

Popular as a snack, this protein-packed food is also a common cause of allergy. Nuts, in fact, share the dubious distinction with fish of being the most commonly implicated in anaphylactic reactions.

Nuts include almonds, Brazil nuts, cashews, coconuts, hazelnuts (filberts), macadamia nuts, nutmeg, peanuts, pecans, pine nuts, pistachios, walnuts and water chestnuts. All are classified as tree nuts except coconuts, peanuts, nutmeg and water chestnuts. Of all the common tree nuts, almonds seem to be the least allergenic. Peanuts, on the other hand, rank toward the top of the allergenic foods list. It is possible that an individual can tolerate peanuts, but be allergic to any tree nut, or vise versa. Still others find they cannot eat any nut.

Approximately one-third of those afflicted with an allergy to peanuts suffer from severe reactions. Super-sensitive individuals can even react to airborne remnants of peanuts and infants have been known to be troubled by the peanut proteins in their mother's milk!

Nuts can be found in such products as candy, cookies, doughnuts, chocolates, ice cream (as well as other frozen desserts), cereals, chili, egg rolls, soups, and margarine—but remnants of some of these things may be inadvertently included in food items that are not intended to contain nuts. The reason for this is that some companies use the same machines to process products that contain nuts as they do for items that don't call for nuts in the recipe, and even the best of cleaning practices may not remove every bit. Likely candidates for this scenario are candy, cookies, dried soups, ice cream, and cereals. As a matter of fact, European chocolates are allowed to be manufactured with leftover chocolate, which might contain nuts—and this may not be disclosed on their label!

This scenario often unfolds in similar ways at home. Foods can pick up traces of nuts when a knife or cutting board is used to chop nuts, and then other foods. By the same token, a scoop can become contaminated when it is used to dip one kind of ice cream without nuts after it is used with one containing nuts. Or a cookie jar can hold remnants from nut-laden cookies that were previously stored there.

Likely symptoms of nut allergies are intestinal discomfort; stuffy nose; asthma; wheezing, skin rashes; tightening of the throat; and itching of the mouth, eye, or ears.

Table 11

Products in which Nuts can be Found

Candy	Ice cream (and other frozen desserts)
Cereals	Margarine
Chili	Pies
Chocolates	Soups
Cookies	Vegetable oil
Doughnuts	Vegetarian burger patties
Egg rolls	

Fish

Seafood has been a favorite for many throughout the years, but for some, it is regarded as anything but a pleasure. More than a few have been known to face violent reactions in the form of anaphylactic shock after eating fish or shellfish. Other less threatening symptoms that have been known to emerge because of an allergy to fish include headaches, stomach aches, tingling in the neck and shoulders, depression and panic attacks.

Proteins called *parvalbumins* contained in seafood are what can often trigger allergic problems. Some may to react to all types of sea dwellers if an allergy exists for any one of the others, whether it be catfish, trout, or salmon; or crustaceans such as shrimp, crab, or lobster; or mollusks such as claims, oysters, or scallops. Usually, if one is allergic to one kind of crustacean, he or she will react to all the other crustaceans. The same holds true for mollusks.

Another problem is that a large volume of seafood has been contaminated with various waste chemicals that are habitually dumped into our rivers, lakes and oceans. These substances could prove to be a culprit in allergy. And if it's your custom to consume canned fish products, there may be additives in tuna and salmon, for instance, that could be potentially allergenic.

Likely you won't find these aquatic creatures as an ingredient in as many processed foods, as with corn, eggs, milk, wheat and nuts. But there are *some*. They include Worcestershire sauce, pasta sauces, Caesar salad dressing and caponata relish, which may contain anchovies. In fact, it is a standard ingredient for Worcestershire sauce.

It is also possible to be unknowingly exposed to fish at restaurants that employ the same oil for French fries as they do for fish. And just as with peanuts, an airborne problem can surface when fish protein finds its way into the air. Some have been known to be affected even after strolling through a fish market!

Table 12

Processed Foods That may or do Contain Seafood	
Caponata relish	Pasta sauces
Caesar salad dressing	Worcestershire sauce

Soy

Of the other foods that have been known to evoke allergic reactions in individuals, soy often poses allergenic problems. Classified as a legume, soybeans are botanically related to peanuts, but the proteins in various legumes differ, which might very well be explain why some who have developed a soy intolerance have no problem with other legumes. Typical symptoms include stuffy nose, intestinal discomfort, bouts of asthma and skin problems. Fortunately, however, allergic reactions are often less severe with soy. Soy may be hiding in baby foods, bread, biscuits, cakes, candy, carob, cereals, ice cream, shortening, thickeners, tofu and vegetable broth.

Chocolate

Chocolate may also be a problem. This popular snack food is known to evoke migraine headaches in sensitive individuals. A substance known as *phenylethylamine*, contained in chocolate, seems to be the culprit because it can dilate the brain's blood vessels. The sugar contained within could also be a problem, as can caffeine. Those allergic to chocolate may also be affected by its relatives cocoa, cola and an ingredient called karaya gum (often listed as "vegetable gum" on product labels).

Yeast

Yeast, a kind of fungus, can also create allergic responses. It is employed as a rising agent in baked goods. It is also a key ingredient in the fermentation process in fermented foods such as vinegar and alcoholic beverages such as beer. And, of course, it's found in breads (including rolls, buscuits, etc.). Sensitivity to yeast, however, it not usually allergy related, although it is possible to develop an allergy to the proteins present there.

Some of the food items that may contain or definitely contain yeast besides those just specifically mentioned are barbecue sauce, buttermilk, cake, cheese, cookies, crackers, dried fruits, grapes, horseradish, ketchup, luncheon meats, mayonnaise, mustard, olives, pasta, pickles, pretzels, relish, salad dressing, sausage, sour cream, tomato sauce and yogurt. A more comprehensive list can be found in table 13.

Table 13

Foods That may or do Contain Yeast

Alcoholic beverages	Mushrooms
Baking mixes	Mustard
Barbecue sauce	Olives
Buttermilk	Pasta
Cake	Pastry
Cheese	Pickles
Chili sauce	Pretzels
Chutney	Relish
Cookies	Root beer
Crackers	Salad dressing
Croutons	Sauerkaut
Dried fruits	Sausage
Enriched flour	Sour cream
Ginger ale	Soy sauce
Grapes	Spice mixes
Horseradish	Stuffing
Kefir	Tea
Ketchup	Tomato sauce
Luncheon meats	Truffles
Malted milk	Vinegars
Marmite or Vegemite	Worcestershire sauce
Mayonnaise	Yogurt
Miso	

Other Foods Containing Caffeine

Other caffeine-laden foods besides chocolate can also pose problems. Coffee, tea and soft drinks are included in this category. One must remember that caffeine is a drug. It has the ability to raise blood pressure, cause the heart to race, create nervousness and force kidneys and adrenal glands to overwork. If nothing more, it is responsible for an untold number of chronic insomnia cases.

Sugar

Refined sugar of every kind has become notorious for causing all kinds of dysfunctions. But it may not be solely responsible for an allergy or even be the cause of it at all in itself. However, its constant presence in the diet is harmful because it displaces nourishing foods that might otherwise be consumed that might help ward off allergies. In addition, sugar may aggravate other food intolerances.

Food Additives

While it may be true that allergies to specific foods are possible, all too often one is fooled into thinking this is so in his or her case, when the problem lies with something with which the food has become adulterated. This has become a serious problem, in fact. There are so many additions to foods today, it just could be that medical science will someday discover that *all* food allergy is caused by one of more of these substances.

There are a slew of additives included that are employed for the purposes of preserving, flavor enhancing, coloring, bleaching, and sweetening. Others are added to aid baked goods to rise evenly or to expedite the processing and preparation of foods. Then there are the chemical residues that remain from pesticide applications. That's not to mention any industrial pollutants that fortuitously work their way into crops via the air, soil or water.

Just some of the more potentially harmful additives are BHA (butylated hydroxyanisole), BHT (butylated hydroxytolune), BVO (brominated vegetable oil), carrageenan, casein and sodium caseinate, dyes, EDTA (ethylenediamine tetraacetate), gum arabic, heptyl paraben, hydrolyzed vegetable protein, mannitol, modified food starch, monoglycerides and diglycerides, MSG (monosodium glutamate), phosphates, propyl gallate, sodium benzoate, sodium carboxymethylcellulose, sodium nitrate and sodium nitrite, sugar, sulfites (including sulfur dioxide and sodium bisulite) and TBHQ (tertiary butylhydroquinone).

The possibilities are almost endless. Sulfur dioxide may be used to preserve the color of dried fruits such as raisins or employed in the production of corn to prevent its fermentation during processing. MSG may be found in potato chips, soups, and many more food items, placed there to enhance flavor. Fresh fish may be laced with sodium nitrite or sodium benzoate to retard spoilage. And it's standard practice to wax produce such as apples and bell peppers to enhance color.

What's more, the matter can be even further complicated when, for instance, one reacts to MSG, when the problem should be blamed on wheat or soy (or something with which the wheat or soy has been contaminated) because this additive is sometimes produced from one of these items. Or when waxed fruit generates allergic symptoms, it may be attribtable to a fungicide used with the wax.

On top of this, labels are not always reliable. Sometimes certain ingredients are substituted by a manufacturers because another ingredient is not available at the time, and this is not specified. Canola oil, for example, may be used instead of corn oil. In some cases a label may read something like: "canola and/or soybean oil," which is somewhat of an improvement, but one still can't tell for sure which one is included or whether both are present. Other labels are misleading. For instance, a coffee creamer marked as "nondairy" may actually contain milk products such as casein, lactose or whey, which in themselves contain ingredients from unexpected sources: corn, beef or pork fat, petrochemicals, etc. Still other labels are ambiguous. For example, the term "sweetener" can mean the product contains corn syrup or that it contains dextrose. A label can be non-specific as well, as when a food contains an egg product under the guise of a term such as "emulsifier."

In addition, unwelcome additives may also find their ways into food in another fashion. Antibiotics such as penicillin and sulfamethazine are often mixed with farm animal feed as a precaution against disease, only to be absorbed by the animal and ultimately result in contaminated meat. Hormones are also used on livestock to speed growth and make for a tenderer product. One may react after ingesting a serving of chicken, never the wiser that the problem was brought on by the penicillin to which he or she is sensitive. Often, these additions can produce violent allergic reactions.

Pesticide Residues

Pesticides come in the form of insecticides (to control insects), miticides (to eliminate mites), herbicides (to kill weeds), rodenticides (to destroy rodents), and fungicides (to inhibit the growth of fungus). Many have proved to be so harmful they have been banned, such as the notorious DDT. Even the mildest of the ones still in use today, however, may pose a big problem for some.

Pesticide residues are found in plant foods and animal products as well (via the food the animals themselves eat). Even an organic gardener's crops may absorb some of the chemical treatment that a nearby neighbor sprays on his or her yard via the air or water.

And speaking about water, it too has been known to be a source of allergy. There is more on it in the chapter that follows.

Chapter 4
Watch Out for Water

Water. Good, reliable H_2O. We drink it, brush our teeth with it, cook with it, and wash with it. Over 60% of the human body's weight is from water and a loss of some 15% will prove fatal. It's a substance vital to all life. So how can anyone be allergic to it? Actually, water allergy (aguagenic urticaria) is very rare. Only a handful of cases have ever been reported.

As is often the case with food, allergic reactions to water occur not from the water itself, but from contaminants *in* the water. Agricultural chemicals and industrial waste is eventually drawn into it to some extent. All sources of water are affected by this; *i. e.*, wells, springs, rivers, ponds, lakes and reservoirs, as well as groundwater. In addition, drinking water from the tap contains additives put there by municipal processing plants.

Tap Water

There are many hundreds of potentially harmful contaminants that inadvertently seep into the water supply. Nitrate is one example. Tap water possesses the same concentrations of this chemical as raw water because conventional purification practices do not remove it. Probably the largest source of contamination originates from nitrogen fertilizers. Other sources are animal waste and inefficient sewage disposal.

Sulfates are another example. The chief sources of these contaminants are manufacturing plants, waste discharges, septic tank systems and rainfall filtering down through rocks. Sulfates possess a laxative effect on the human body and a sensitive individual can experience diarrhea after an innocent drink.

Lead can also pose problems. It reaches the water via manufacturers of storage batteries, bearings, and the like, as well as from landfills. Children are affected by much lower levels of this metal than adults.

Other potential hazards come in the form of benzene, a by-product of petroleum manufacturing; trichloroethylene (TCE), found in numerous household products and employed as an industrial degreasing agent; and chloroform, used widely in industry.

Then there are the pesticides. And that names only a few.

In addition, tap water is usually the victim of the additives chlorine and fluoride. Chlorine is used to reduce microbial hazards and fluoride is employed to retard tooth decay. The matter is worsened when chlorine is put to use in this regard, because it combines with other substances to form chloroform and additional by-products. In fact, these by-products can be formed right at the kitchen sink because chlorine vapors can escape into the air and combine with it when water is running from the tap, especially if it is hot. Not only can this be a problem for sensitive individuals *drinking* the water, but also for some who are *breathing* the air near it.

Then there are further possibilities. Lead can leach into the water from household plumbing connectors. Perchloroethylene (PCE), or tetrachloroethylene, which is used in the lining of water distribution pipes composed of cement, can also make its way into tap water.

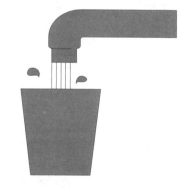

There are many hundreds of potentially harmful contaminants that sneak into tap water.

Table 14

Common Water Pollutants	
Arsenic	Lead
Barium	Mercury
Benzene	Methoxychlor
Cadmium	Nitrates
Carbon tetrachloride	Selenium
Chlorine	Sulfates
Chromium	Toxaphene
Endrin	Trichloroethylene
Fluoride	Vinyl chloride
Landane	

Bottled Water

Some allergic individuals might find salvation in bottled water. But even it often does not escape some of these contaminants, whether it be labeled as "spring," "sparkling," "mineral," "still," "distilled" or just plain "drinking water." And the addition of carbonation in some varieties has no bearing on this. Tests have been known to reveal the presence of benzene, PCE, toluene, chloroform and number of other pollutants in various samples. Often, the concentrations fall below maximum contamination levels set for public water supplies. But that does not mean there wouldn't be enough to produce allergic symptoms in sensitive individuals.

The are several avenues whereby contaminants can enter bottled water. The bottler may fail to remove all the pollutants from the raw water. They can be accidentally added by the bottler. Or sometimes the container itself can leach contaminants into the product—especially if it is made of plastic, which most of them are.

Symptoms that may arise as a result of taking in contaminants from drinking water are many and include diarrhea, nausea, bloating, mouth ulcers, asthma and even hay fever. If you have an allergy and have tried everything else, perhaps your answer could be found in the water you drink. But even if you are not reacting to the chemicals there, you may still be finding some of these substances troublesome in another way. There are countless chemicals used everyday, any one of which could pose a problem. Let's take a hard look at them in the next chapter.

Chapter 5
Household Chemical Concerns

There has been a greater concern over the growing use of household chemicals over the last few years than ever before. It's no wonder. These substances can add a considerable burden to the environment, particularly indoors.

On the list are cleaners and related products, such as those used for dishwashing, laundry, ovens, toilets, bathtubs, sinks, drains, carpets and upholstery, and those utilized for polishing furniture and waxing floors; personal care products such as deodorants, hair conditioners, hair sprays, nail polish, perfumes, mascara, lipstick, colognes, shampoos, lotions, shaving cream, toothpaste, mouthwash, and soap; and home improvement items, including paint, paint thinners, stains, varnishes, glues, and sealers.

Cleaning chemicals are a serious offender—a harsh irony, as they are used to clean up dirt and other contaminants, not contribute to them. Because of the job they have been specifically designed to do, they seem the most innocuous of any other category of substances. Yet, as with most products, we tend to use them liberally—and

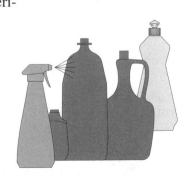

There are numerous household chemicals that can trigger allergic symptoms.

they contain some strong ingredients, such as ammonia, bleach, chlorine, phosphates, and sometimes volatile petroleum solvents in the form of acetone, benzene, naptha, toluene and xylene.

Cleaning Chemicals and Related Products

Aerosols

Any product dispensed from an aerosol container can be especially troublesome, not just because of the solvents and volatile chemical mixtures, but also because of the propellants that must be used to dispatch these chemicals. Typical propellants are propane, butane, isobutane, pentane, nitrous oxide and methylene chloride. A significant portion of such chemicals, as well as the other contents, are released to evaporate into the air every time the product is used. It is estimated that as much as 15 pounds of propellant is released in the average household annually.

Oven Cleaners

Oven cleaners may very well be one of the worst household pollutants of this category because they are especially potent. They have to be in order to adequately take care of all those burned-on food drippings from meat sauces, pies and what-have-you that have been left to accumulate for months. Oven cleaners contain such substances as hydroxethyl cellulose, sodium hydroxide (lye) and polyoxyethylene fatty ethers.

Drain Cleaners

Drain cleaners also pose a serious problem. Their ingredients include trichloroethane, petroleum distillates and sodium hydroxide (of which the product is almost entirely composed). Sometimes ammonia is an ingredient. Allergies aside, ammonia forms the deadly gas chloramine if mixed with a chlorine-based cleanser or bleach.

Bathroom and Kitchen Cleaners

These cleaning agents are strong too, containing such substances as phosphates and chlorine bleach. Toilet bowl disinfectants can be especially potent.

Laundry Detergents

Some have been bothered by clothing detergents, not so much during the application process but long afterward, when the clean apparel is worn. Phosphates or other chemicals leave residues in garments and can be inhaled by the wearer all day long or remain in constant contact with the skin surface, leaving plenty of opportunity for more sensitive individuals to succumb to.

On top of this, detergents and soaps enhance other allergies because they break down keratin, the protein compound of skin, as well as the protective oils residing on the skin surface. This leaves the skin wide open for other allergenic substances that can, as a result, be more rapidly absorbed.

Furniture Polish and Floor Wax

Furniture polish is another widely used item that deserves mention. It contains chemicals such as chlorine, phenols, acrylics, formaldehyde—and sometimes even pesticides. Floor wax also contains many of the same ingredients and other volatile chemicals as furniture polish. These substances can emit vapors for lengthy periods of time and come in contact with the skin quite easily.

Personal Care Products

Lipstick

Actually, lipstick should be regarded as a food because a lot of it is taken orally—in effect, it is eaten. Women inadvertantly lick it off over time in the process of talking and eating. That's the reason they commonly renew it several times during the course of every day. By then they have ingested the chemicals of which it is composed, in the form of dyes, waxes, oils and perfumes.

Antiperspirants and Deodorants

How can these products be a problem? An antiperspirant's job is to defeat, albeit temporarily, the body's ability to perspire. The chemicals employed for this purpose actually produce a slight irritation to the underarm skin that swells the openings of the sweat glands and blocks the excretion of perspiration. This can in turn create additional irritation that is more severe. Sometimes outright infection is the result. Deodorants work in a different way. They contain substances that both attack odor-producing bacteria and mask body odor. Many of these chemicals serve as allergens to the sensitive.

Underarm deodorants and antiperspirants are composed of such substances as aluminum chlorohydrate, alcohol and fragrances. They also contain bactericides, some of which have been known to cause health problems.

Nail Care Products

Nail polish and nail polish remover are of particular concern because their vapors are particularly potent before they have dried. The solvents of which nail polish is composed include toluene, butyl acetate, ethyl acetate and amyl acetate. These substances can even produce a narcotic effect if inhaled in large quantities and they play havoc with the nervous system. The removers contain acetone or a close chemical cousin. They are highly volatile substances, and can therefore be readily taken into the respiratory system. In fact, they are potent enough to dissolve not only nail polish, but ball-point pens, plastic jewelry, and other plastic items. The inhalation of acetone can produce headaches, fatigue, bronchial irritation and even unconsciousness. And certainly this creates lots of potential for skin irritations.

Cuticle removers and softeners also deserve a word. They are probably the harshest of the cosmetics products. Most contain either potassium hydroxide or sodium hydroxide. As a result, the pH level is about as much as a drain cleaner!

Perfumes and Colognes

These items are also composed of potent and volatile chemicals. A single scent may include as many as 200 ingredients. The olfactory senses readily adapt to any fragrance or odor, and once applied, the consumer will forget its there, and will continue to breath its vapors, some of which will be absorbed by the skin. Minute amounts can be transferred to others from close contact. Even this minor displacement has been known to initiate severe symptoms in some and has been responsible for convincing a few that they had actually become allergic to their spouse or other family member.

Hair Care Products

Hair spray can be, at the least, an allergic threat to some. About 25% of hair sprays contain methylene chloride, sometimes disguised on the label as "aromatic hydrocarbons." Furthermore, some sprays may contain polyvinyl pyrrolidone (PVP). Shellac or ethyl cellulose is often included to make PVP more resistant to moisture, and plasticizers such as benzyl alcohol (derived from toluene) are also added to make the PVP more flexible. It has been noted that immediately after exposure to hair sprays, there is a measurable reduction in a person's ability to exhale.

Hair dyes are another source of concern for those who have become chemically susceptible. Most of the dyes today are synthetic and contain additives that serve as oxidizers, color modifiers, stabilizers, and the like. One substance, aminophenol, is used in orange-red and medium brown dyes. The inhalation of this chemical may produce asthma. Another common skin allergen that may be included in dyes is paraphenylenediamine. It can cross-react with dyes in foods or medications.

Even shampoos, which may contain formaldehyde and other strong chemicals, can be a menace to the sensitive.

Mascara

These and similar products also contain chemicals that could become allergens to many, even those labeled "hypoallergenic" (although the chance in this case is less likely). The eyelids are particularly sensitive, actually the most sensitive area of the face as well as that of the entire body. They possess a strong tendency to react to substances applied to and around them.

Toothpaste and Mouthwash

These two items can also present problems for some. They contain a number of chemicals, including pyrophosphates, dyes, benzoic acid and formaldehyde. Symptoms that are produced from short-term formaldehyde exposure alone include skin rashes, burning eyes, runny nose, sore throat, dry cough and nausea.

Home Improvement Items

Paints and Related Supplies

Paints can be especially bad as they may contain as many as 300 toxic materials, including acetone, benzene, cadmium, formaldehyde, naphtha, and toluene. Paint removers are worse. They contain not only benzene and toluene, but chemicals such as acetone, ethyl ether and turpentine. Stains, varnishes and glue also contain some of these chemicals.

Other Chemical Concerns

Children's school supplies and play items, as innocent as they may seem, have been known to produce allergies too. Crayons, paste, finger paints and clay are included.

Other problematic substances exist in the form of pool chemicals. Chlorine, muriatic acid, stabilizers and algae growth depressants emit strong vapors and can be hard on skin.

Still other items that fall into the household chemical category are the air fresheners. Whether aerosol or ornamental, their job is to rid the air of bad odors, and that they do—but in the process, they add their own chemical contaminants to the air, among which can include cresol, ethanol (ethyl alcohol), propylene glycol morpholine and form-aldehyde.

These are just some of the chemical products found around the home that can trigger allergies, with one major exception—that of pesticides. They will be covered next.

Table 15

Common Household Products that can Generate Allergies

After-shave lotions	Mascara
Air fresheners	Metal cleaners
Bathroom cleaners	Mouthwash
Bubble baths	Nail polish
Carpet cleaners	Nail polish remover
Colognes	Oven cleaners
Contact lense cleaner	Paint
Deodorants	Paint remover
Dishwasher detergents	Paint thinners
Dishwashing liquids	Perfumes
Drain cleaners	Pool chemicals
Eye shadow	Rouge
Fabric softeners	Sealers
Face creams	Shampoos
Floor wax	Shaving cream
Furniture polish	Shoe polish
Glass cleaners	Soap
Glue	Spot removers
Hair conditioners	Stains
Hair sprays	Toothpaste
Laundry detergents	Upholstery cleaner
Lipstick	Varnish
Lotions	Varnish remover

Chapter 6
Those Persistent Pesticides

Pesticides certainly deserve deep concern when it comes to health. They are usually blamed for serious illness and have been responsible for a number of accidental deaths. But they too cannot be ruled out as a potential allergen.

At any rate, pesticides are tough stuff. They are poisons intended to destroy specific forms of life, which makes them anything but harmless. Although containers clearly display cautions regarding their application, many are far too casual about dispensing them. Even when extreme care is taken, it is not always enough. When applied out-of-doors on a lawn or garden, pesticide residues can be picked up by shoes or a roaming pet only to be deposited inside and/or the wind can carry them places they weren't intended to go. Once pesticides have been applied inside, it is very difficult, and sometimes impossible, to completely remove them.

Just a few of the active ingredients that are found in household pesticides are toxaphene, mercury, dinitrophenol, bendiocarb, phenol methylcarbonate, tolumide, and arsenic compounds. That's not to consider the inert ingredients, which are not always disclosed on the label and can actually be more toxic to the body than the active ingredients.

Pesticides pose a threat both as an airborne allergen or as a contact allergen. The symptoms are many, any of which could be considered an allergic reaction. Included are respiratory difficulties, blurred vision, twitching, mental confusion, digestive disturbances, headaches, weakness, dizziness, depression, and anxiety.

Pesticides often Overlooked

Before leaving the subject, it had better be said that there are obscure examples of pesticides found in and around the home. Most think of pesticides as sprays to be applied to lawns, trees and bushes, or areas inside where insects are spotted. But some pesticides are often overlooked or aren't recognized as such. Mothballs are a prime example. They are usually desposited and forgotten. Not only do they contaminate closets and to a certain extent the rest of the house, but their vapors are absorbed by clothes and other items. Mothballs are made up of paradichlorobenzene and naphthalene. Among other things, they have been known to cause headaches, asthma attacks, rapid heartbeats and depression.

Insect repellents are not to be overlooked either. Even they can prove to be a problem, especially those containing diethyl-toluamide (deet).

Pest strips, as well as flea and tick collars and powders, count too. They all contain a wide variety of insecticides. In the case of strips and collars, these insecticides are gradually released from the plastic to permeate the air, possibly to affect both the animal and its master. The administration of powder, of course, can dispense its share of toxic particulate matter not only in the air, but on the skin. It too can affect the human being as well as the pet.

Speaking of pets, they can also unfortunately lie at the root of an allergy. Next let's take a closer look at this scenario.

Table 16

Pesticides or Pesticide-Laden Items often Overlooked in the Home	
Flea and tick collars	Mothballs
Flea powders	Pest strips
Insect repellents	

Chapter 7
The Thing About Pets

Domestic animals are extremely popular as pets. Over 100 million in the United States are kept for this purpose. Although they can provide pleasure, ease tension and promote love, there's no telling how many sneezes, runny noses, itchy eyes and other symptoms have been brought on by their hair, dander and feathers.

Dogs

As far as our furry friends are concerned, dogs make one of the largest hair and dander contributions. The dandruff is especially bad for sensitive individuals because it can easily break down into tiny flakes that can readily enter nasal passages. In addition, it absorbs sebum, the oily substance that is secreted by the dog's sebaceous glands, which itself has been known to initiate allergic symptoms. For that matter, as with other kinds of animals, even the urine can be an allergen.

Still, many have been affected by the hair. As in the case of other such animals, the protein matter of the hair shaft, largely keratin (not actually the hair itself), is what allergists point to as the instigator of health problems. There is room for argument, however, because the hair is also coated with sebum—and this makes it easy for other matter to cling to the hair as well. The hair itself is too large to be inhaled, but the foregoing offers a number of possibilities for those who pet dogs to develop skin allergies, adults and children alike. Also, those who do not contact the animal may still be affected by encounters with stray hairs.

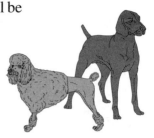

And whether Chihuahua or poodle, cocker spaniel or German Shepherd, short-haired or long-haired, there is no hard evidence that any one breed is more prone to produce allergies. However, it is possible for an individual to be affected by just one breed. Some dogs, such as poodles, may produce somewhat less of a plight in the sense that they shed

No breed of dog is any less prone to produce allergies than another.

less, therefore leaving less hair behind, but in an allergic sense, their hair is no different than any other dog's.

Common symptoms of dog allergy are rhinitis, asthma and eczema.

Cats

Cats are generally worse offenders for those predisposed to allergies. Their hair, finer and softer than a dog's, sheds more readily, making more of it available to the air and carrying with it a variety of foreign matter that is potentially allergenic. Moreover, there is an allergen in the saliva of a cat that gets deposited on the coat during grooming. Both the hair and dander, which also contain sebum, tend to linger in the air or become attached indefinitely to home furnishing, such as stuffed furniture, curtains and carpeting—and they can certainly cling to clothes.

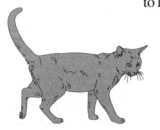

Some severely sensitive people have been known to experience an allergy attack even when entering a room or building in which a cat had previously been an occupant. Up to 30% of those with chronic respira-

The saliva of a cat contains an allergen that gets deposited on the coat during grooming.

tory problems, particularly asthma, have been found to have an allergy to cats.

Unlike those of dogs, breeds with longer hair have a tendency to be more allergenic than the others. It is possible for one to be allergic to only one breed, just as in the case of dogs. Interestingly, female cats have a tendency to pose less of an allergy problem than male cats and the males seem to be even less allergenic if neutered. Also, one study revealed that dark-haired cats seen to evoke more severe symptoms in their allergic masters than the light-colored variety.

In addition, cat allergens can cross-react with those of dogs. So if you decide to give up your cat and plan to substitute a dog for it, beware.

As with a dog, typical symptoms of cat allergy include rhinitis, asthma and eczema.

Horses

Horses can also initiate allergic reactions in people. Although it is unlikely that a horse will be found around the house, stables and barns are another thing. As many as 19% of allergic patients are sensitive to horse allergens. The usual resulting ailment is asthma. Some are so sensitive to this kind of animal that even being exposed to horse manure, as in a garden, can set off a reaction, as can furniture stuffed with horsehair and the allergen-laden clothes of someone who has been riding a horse. Such sensitive individuals are also often allergic to similar animals such as mules, donkeys and zebras.

Birds

Of course, our feathered friends cannot be overlooked as a potential allergy problem. Bird feathers fraught with dander and attached to the oily portion of the skin have proved particularly bothersome to many. Canaries, parrots, parakeets, myna birds and pigeons are just some of the examples. Not only can a child be besieged with constant respiratory problems because of a pet parakeet in his or her bedroom, but a farmer can be affected with a flare-up of sinusitis every time he goes into his henhouse, or an elderly gentleman might suffer an asthma attack after his daily routine of feeding pigeons in the park. One report related that a woman's asthma was caused by sparrows that had been nesting in vines beneath her bedroom window.

Feather particles and dander are not the only trouble with birds. Minute particles from the feces and nasal secretions of birds such as those of parakeets and pigeons have been known to trigger allergic responses. Not only can this result in rhinitis and asthma, but more serious diseases can develop. Hypersensitivity pneumonitis (involving inflammation of alveolar walls and bronchioles) is one example, as is bird-fancier's lung (extrinsic allergic alveolitis). It might be added that birds are also capable of transmitting psittacosis (better known as parrot fever).

It might also be added that some of those with allergies to birds can develop a cross-reaction to egg proteins and therefore react adversely when eating eggs.

Other Animals

There are many other animals that can precipitate an allergic attack, most likely from their skin particles or proteins from their urine. Examples include rabbits, gerbils, hamsters, guinea pigs, ferrets and mice. And these don't have to be pets, per se. Those working in research labs are vulnerable from exposure to guinea pigs, rats, mice or monkeys. By the same token, veterinarians, zoo workers, farmers, circus performers, animal breeders and pet shop employees can fall victim to allergy as well.

In addition, one cannot dismiss the allergens that may crop up because of a more exotic pet. Aquariums can harbor mold and algae, and dust from snake or reptile tanks can be troublesome as well.

Other Considerations

An allergy to pets can sometimes be difficult to pin down. Symptoms may emerge at any time. Sometimes, in fact, they may not surface for years because it requires a longer period of time for some to develop a sensitivity. In fact, according to Fort Worth allergist Normand Tremblay, a person may experience low-grade symptoms for a long time that are too subdued to regard as consequential. He goes on to say, "If you have constant daily exposure to pet dander, you do develop some allergic immunity on your own to the allergen. That means you won't have immediate reactions to the allergen, but you could still have chronic low-grade symptoms that you may consider a normal part of day-to-day life."

A person who suspects an allergy to a dog or cat, no matter when it may surface, may have been deceived anyway. As mentioned previously, he or she could be reacting to a flea collar or flea powder. A medication for mange or another ailment that has been applied to the animal's coat could also be a culprit. In addition, an animal that is allowed to roam freely could be exposing itself to pollen, pesticide residues, or other potential allergens without the owner's knowledge.

Animal hair, feather, or dander can haunt allergy victims in another way. One, for instance, may suffer from sinus discomfort after sleeping on a feather pillow or wearing clothes made from down.

Table 17

Potential Allergens Associated with Animals	
Dander	Saliva
Feathers	Sebum
Hair	Urine

Hopefully, you now have a good idea about how animals can enter into the allergy scene, but they are not the only living creatures that can trigger allergic attacks. Insects can also be guilty. Let's consider them next.

Chapter 8
Those Pesky Insects

The bite from a mosquito or sting from a bee is only a minor annoyance for most people. At worst, after the initial surprise, the skin in the affected area forms a red welt, and perhaps an intense itch of short duration follows.

For allergic individuals, the matter is quite different. The territory around a bite or sting may swell and that swelling may persist. Skin irritation may advance beyond the affected area. More widespread symptoms may show their ugly face, such as sneezing, wheezing or itching and swelling around the eyes. More severe symptoms can come in the form of hoarseness; difficulty in swallowing, breathing or speaking; vomiting; rapid heartbeat, and confusion. In some of the less fortunate allergy victims, anaphylactic shock results.

Some individuals are racked not only with an immediate reaction but a second one as well that may be delayed for as much as 2 weeks. Typical symptoms include fever, headaches, joint pain, hives and malaise.

Reactions to multiple stings or bites can include fever, headache, swelling, diarrhea, drowsiness and even convulsions and unconsciousness.

Stinging insects are worst than the biting kinds because they generate more severe reactions. They include bees, wasps, hornets, yellow jackets, and scorpions (which actually fall under the scientific classification *scorpionida*, rather than the class known as *insecta*, the label for insects). Insect venom is injected via stingers attached to the rear sections.

Biting insects come in the form of flies, fleas, mosquitoes, bed-bugs and ants—although some species of ants, such as the fire ant, do sting. Spiders can be included in the category of biters, although scientifically they are classified as mites and don't actually belong to the insect family. The venom of the biters is conveyed via the saliva.

Bees

There are some 12,000 species of bees. This includes such varieties as the bumblebee, carpenter bee, cuckoo bee and honeybee. Many are important to the pollination process and the honeybee is instrumental in the production of honey and beeswax. They vary in coloring as well as behavior. Some are more aggressive and others, such as the honeybee and bumblebee, are not. These particularly easy-going breeds will not likely sting unless disturbed. But the venom of any can evoke allergic reaction.

The venom of bees varies in potency from species to species, so some may cause more severe reactions than others. In addition, the concentrations of venom can vary with the different seasons. Anyone allergic to bees will likely react to wasps and ants as well.

Wasps, Hornets and Yellow Jackets

These insects are generally more aggressive than bees and individuals are therefore more likely to get pricked by one. Some, in fact, have been known to sting without being provoked. Their venom is similar that of bees. Hornets and yellow jackets can also bite.

Scorpions

Most scorpions prefer retreat rather than fight and don't usually sting unless molested. Symptoms produced from a sting vary from species to species. They may include swelling, sweating, stomach ache, vomiting, numbness, chest pain, respiratory distress, salivation and convulsions. Stings can prove fatal in some cases, especially when certain species are involved.

Ants

There are approximately 15,000 species of ants. Any of them can cause distress to the allergic sensitive. Of this number, the fire ant poses the most serious problem. Residing in the southeasten portion of the United States, these insects, when threatened, attack aggressively in voluminous numbers. They may be red in color as well as black, brown, yellow or orange and have a way of blending into the landscape. They can be found in yards, parks, vacant lots or just about anywhere.

Their stings burn intensely and the symptoms produced by their venom, which contains toxic oily alkaloids, is different than those caused by other insect stings. At first, only a welt can be seen. But hours later, blister-like sacs appear on the skin. This is replaced by pus as the fluid inside the sacs drains away. The day after the sting, the wound becomes surrounded by swelling or a red circle. The affected area then usually crusts over. The entire affair may go on for as long as a week or more. Such stings can prove fatal to particularly sensitive individuals.

Furthermore, one is more likely to receive multiple stings, because unlike the bee, which dies after it does its damage, the fire ant is capable of repeated stings.

Flies

Flies that commonly produce allergic symptoms in the U. S. are black flies, biting midges and deerflies.

Black flies (also known as turkey gnats or buffalo gnats in some regions) are probably the worst. They are so aggressive as to bite through clothing if need be and they are capable of initiating anaphylactic shock.

Biting midges (also known as moose flies, sand flies and gnats) are discouraged easily by the wind, probably because of their small size, but they can be a nuisance on still days.

Deerflies customarily make deer, cattle and horses their victims, but human beings are not always overlooked by them. Unfortunately, they are wicked biters and widespread symptoms can be generated.

Fleas

Fleas, which feed exclusively on blood, are renown for making dogs and cats miserable, but they do likewise to birds and other animals. There are a number of different varieties, including the cat flea, the chicken flea, the rat flea and the chigoe flea, not to mention the human flea. The human flea does not necessarily confine its activities to people any more than the other types make animals their only host. The chigoe flea, in fact, is a well-known human pest in the tropics. Fleas can produce allergies in both people and pets.

Mosquitos

It doesn't matter that these insects are smaller in size than flies and many other insects. They can still create their share of trouble. Bites generally cause short-term itching for the typical person, but those who are sensitive can be struck with swelling, hives, dizziness, headaches, and the like. The problem originates with the saliva the mosquito injects along with the bite, which can contain allergens. The female of the species are the biters. And they are easily identifiable because the beating of their wings produces that familiar high-pitched noise that makes one instinctively swat the air.

Bedbugs

Bedbugs (*Cimex lectularius*) often find homes inside mattresses, or between the mattress and box springs. These brown insects resemble tiny lentils—flat and oval in shape—and are approximately a quarter-inch long. They emerge during the nighttime hours to feed on human blood. A bite will most likely not make you ill since bedbugs do not carry disease, but they can be a big time problem for those allergic to them. A bite for the particularly sensitive is capable of producing anaphylaxis.

Spiders

These eight-legged, multi-eyed creatures—of which there are some 30,000 species—are abundant worldwide. All spiders possess venom glands but only a few are harmful to everyone, such as the black widow and brown recluse spider. Any bite by a spider, however, can result in an allergic reaction to those so sensitive. Unless by accident, spiders don't bite except when provoked.

Table 18

Insects and Other Small Forms of Life Regarded as such that can Trigger Allergies	
Ants	Mosquitoes
Bees	Scorpions
Fleas	Spiders
Flies	Wasps

Other Stings

Although not regarded as an insect by an stretch, the jellyfish also deserves mention. This marine animal is armed with nematocysts (stinging cells) that are intended to sting and paralyze its prey, but it packs a powerful punch to the human organism. The venom of some jellyfish can even cause death.

Other Matters to Consider

It's true one may allergically react to an insect bite or sting, but it might not be because of the venom coursing through their bloodstream. No one has an idea about where a particular attacking insect has been. If a wasp, for instance, has been exposed to insecticide (and not yet been affected by it), it might be the poison intended for the insect itself that is troubling you.

Or for that matter, an insect might be exposed to any number of other contaminants that could be transmitted in minuscule amounts to a sensitive individual through not only a bite or sting, but merely by being in direct contact. This could apply to non-stinging, non-biting insects as well.

Also it must be pointed out that some individuals develop allergies to the body parts of insects as well as their saliva and/or feces. This number may be as high as 30% for cockroaches alone. Such a situation can be of particular concern in certain portions of the country where annual swarms take place.

And one final word. A drug might be implicated in the case of an insect bite or sting. Almost one-third of those with allergies to insects also have allergic reactions to drugs.

Not only can people develop allergies to the bite or sting of an insect, but to its body parts or excrements as well.

That takes care of the insects. Now let's examine another possible trigger of allergies—plants.

Chapter 9

The Problem with Plants

It's an established fact that pollen manufactured from weeds, grasses and trees can be an allergen. And even the kind of plants producing beautiful flowers cannot be excluded from the list of allergens. Granted, flower pollen will not likely be a problem in most cases as previously stated, but it should be noted that the chrysanthemum is related to ragweed, one of the worst culprits for provoking allergies. If you are allergic to ragweed, you might also react to chrysanthemums.

But no matter what kind of plant pollen is involved or suspected of being involved in an allergy, one could be reacting to a pesticide or industrial pollutant that has been absorbed by that plant.

Poison Ivy, Poison Oak and Poison Sumac

Allergy in relation to pollen is only one matter, however, but what about reactions generated from direct contact with a plant, particularly if it falls under the category of poisonous? Poison ivy, poison oak and poison sumac are particularly intense allergens, so much so that resulting symptoms can continue to spread long after an initial encounter. Even then, there are some that go unaffected after making contact with these plants.

For those less fortunate, itching results, followed by severe skin inflammation that can lead to blistering. An encounter with one of these plants has been known to prove fatal to young children. The toxic substance responsible, urushiol, is created in the liquid of the resin ducts of the leaves, fruit, and flowers, as well as the bark of the stems and roots. However, it does not turn up in the pollen grains.

Unfortunately, it does not require direct contact to cause reactions. The urushiol can be transported from the plants via shoes, clothing, garden tools, and animals, for example, and be picked up by a sensitive person. In fact, poisoning has been known to occur in those who have worn clothes that had been in contact with urushiol a year previously. This substance can even be carried aloft from burning plants, and in this state, it is toxic.

Other Poisonous Plants

There are other poisonous plants capable of producing reactions as well. Poisonwood, found in Florida and the West Indies, is similar to poison ivy. Contact with any portion of this tree—particularly the sap—can cause a rash, blisters, and black skin. Smoke from a burning tree is especially irritating and can not only cause illness, but temporary blindness as well.

Spurge nettle is another example. Immediately after contact, itching and stinging results, followed by a rash. The toxin contained within the plant is conveyed by its tiny hairs.

There are others, such as strophanthus, which is so powerful it is used as an arrow poison. But that advances beyond the scope of allergies.

Table 19

Poisonous Plants that Can Produce Allergic Symptoms	
Poison ivy	Poisonwood
Poison oak	Spurge nettle
Poison sumac	

That's it on the subject of plants. Now let's take a look at how medications affect the allergic sensitive.

Chapter 10
Medicinal Woes

The majority of drugs are synthetic and most contain petrochemical derivatives. Over-the-counter shelves are filled with them, whether it be cough medicines, headache remedies, cold tablets, laxatives, antihistamines, decongestants, sleeping aids, painkillers, antiseptics or salves. And that does not count the vast number of prescription drugs, not to mention those that are illegal.

Medication has often been used as a remedy to alleviate symptoms brought on by allergies. However, the big irony is that some drugs can actually produce allergies in the first place. In fact, 25% of the adverse reactions from drugs are discovered to be allergic in nature.

The remainder fall under the category of side effects. It is an established fact that medications—both over-the-counter and prescription—create numerous side effects. But unlike allergic reactions, side effects are symptoms brought on from the drugs that medical science has learned to expect. They produce prominent reactions with little delay and are clearly described on the labels as well as widely publicized on radio and television.

It's the unanticipated symptoms, however, that are tagged as allergic responses. They don't usually surface for 7 to 10 days after the drug is taken. Subsequent doses can then evoke an immediate—and possibly severe—response, no matter how small these doses may be.

An allergic response can also take place from a dose of medication after one has had a prior exposure to a chemically related substance. The symptoms most likely to occur (whether the medication is swallow, injected or applied topically) involve the skin: itching, hives, rashes, swelling and scaling. One may also become photosensitive; that is, certain drugs may react with sunlight to form allergy-producing substances in the skin. This also makes one more susceptible to sunburn. That's the reason patients are sometimes warned to stay out of the sun when taking certain medications. Other symptoms may include any other reaction generally associated with allergies.

Treatments applied topically are the most apt to produce adverse reactions than those that are taken orally. On the other hand, a drug that is injected is more prone to generate an immediate and severe reaction because it enters the system rapidly.

Penicillin

Of the most troublesome drugs, penicillin heads the list. This widely prescribed antibiotic is used for the treatment of bacterial infections, either killing the bacteria or halting its growth by destroying its cell walls. There are different kinds of penicillins for different kinds of infections and one kind cannot usually be interchanged with another.

Physicians report that from 1% to 10% of the population is allergic to penicillin. Most reactions, however, are mild. Rarely are symptoms severe and in only a few instances a dose has proven fatal.

Antibiotics such as penicillin may produce a delayed allergic reaction for a most ironic reason. When destroying the bacteria causing an infection, they may also kill off beneficial bacteria, enabling other more hardy microorganisms to eventually enter the gut lining and allow allergens to leak into the bloodstream.

Allergic symptoms include itching, swelling, rashes, chills, fever, respiratory distress, peeling skin, muscle aches, joint pain and malaise.

Aspirin

Aspirin (acetylsalicylic acid, or ASA), probably the most widely used drug, is the second most likely medicine to generate allergies. It is prescribed for relieving mild to moderate pain and inflammation, to reduce fever, and to serve as an anticoagulant (blood thinner). As with other drugs, it usually affects the skin, resulting in hives. Other symptoms that sometimes surface include runny nose, stomach aches, vomiting and diarrhea. Aspirin has also been known to cause asthma. In fact, it is best avoided by all asthmatics.

It is not uncommon for those allergic to aspirin to be allergic to other pain relievers or to unrelated drugs. And those allergic to aspirin often react adversely to certain foods or to airborne matter such as mold or pollen. Those with nasal polyps, as well as asthmatics, are more apt to allergically react to aspirin.

Aspirin can be found in a number of over-the-counter medicines used for pain relief, such as headaches and backaches, as well as remedies for sinusitis, upset stomachs and menstrual discomfort. The generic names of aspirin and aspirin-like drugs include aloxiprin, benorylate, choline magnesium trisalicylate, diflunisal and salsalate.

Sulfonamides

Sulfonamides, along with penicillin and aspirin, account for the vast majority of all allergic drug reactions. First introduced in 1932, they belong to the general family of medications referred to as anti-infectives, their purpose being to aid the body in overcoming infections. They destroy bacteria and certain fungi by interfering with their metabolic processes, and are particularly effective for urinary tract infections. Some kinds are used for specific purposes. Triple sulfa, for instance, is prescribed only for vaginal infections. Anyone allergic to sulfa drugs will probably react to any drug chemically related to them. These prescription drugs are a good example of ones that can induce photosensitivity.

Flu Shots

Vaccines designed for the purpose of preventing flu can be a problem for some unlucky people. Not only is there no guarantee flu vaccines will be effective, they are produced from influenza virus cultures and are grown on eggs. Traces of egg sometimes adhere to the virus, despite the fact that the vaccines are highly purified. Those who are allergic to eggs, therefore, may suffer reactions from a flu shot.

Measles vaccines also are included in this, although the risk of adverse reaction is lower.

Allergy Shots

It's a harsh irony, but sometimes allergy shots themselves can create allergic reactions, occasionally even anaphylactic shock! Anaphylaxis occurs if a patient's immune system has not kept pace with the gradual increase in levels of the allergen administered by the physician. Rather than becoming less sensitive to the allergen, the body takes exception to the increased dosage. On occasion, a milder reaction from the preceding treatment heralds this occurrence.

Skin Medications

Ointments used to clear up allergenic skin irritations may not turn out to be your salvation but prolong the problem instead. Preservatives such as ethyenediamine, parabens and mercury, which are often included in them, are a common cause of allergy itself!

Illegal Drugs

Drugs purchased on the street deserve a word too. As bad as they are in themselves, marijuana can cause dryness of the mouth, nausea, diarrhea, respiratory distress, inflamed eyelids and spasms. If it is smoked, all the worse. Amphetamines can trigger rashes and asthma, as can cocaine. Barbiturates can cause rashes and blisters around the mouth.

Other Problems to Consider

As in other cases of allergy, one may be convinced he or she is allergic to certain medications, but is not. The culprit could be hidden in the drug. Just as with food, medicines contain additives. They are included as preservatives, colorings, flavorings, excipients (binders), lubricants, and such. These ingredients can number in the dozens and don't usually turn up on labels. Even vitamins are not excluded.

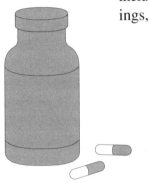

For example, sodium benzoate may be employed as a preservative in a headache remedy, tartrazine (a yellow dye) might be used to color a sleeping pill or calcium stearate could be an ingredient serving as a lubricant for a multiple vitamin. Foods can be involved as well. Some who are allergic to wheat may find that they can't take pharmaceuticals that contain wheat.

Just as with food, medicines contain additives that can produce allergies.

Table 20
Medications Most Likely to Trigger Allergies
Aspirin Penicillin Sulfonamides

Some figure they can find a safe haven in biological drugs, those that are made from natural sources. But they too contain preservatives.

If you don't have an allergy to medications, nor to anything thus far mentioned, still something else may be the cause. Let's examine those possibilities next.

Chapter 11
Other Culprits

As can be seen, allergies can certainly emerge from unexpected sources. What follows are more examples of this nature, some of which you may suspect, some of which are quite surprising. If your allergic problem ranks among the more unusual, you may spot the answer here.

Clothing

Clothes in themselves can be a threat to the allergic. How so? When new, most all apparel is treated with substances that serve as shrink-proofing, waterproofing, mothproofing and wrinkle-proofing, as well as functioning as mildew resistors, stain repellents and static inhibitors. Formaldehyde is one of the most common used. There is no guarantee, either, that this chemical can be eliminated with repeated washings. This can also hold true for sheets and other bedding, and other items made of cloth such as handkerchiefs.

Synthetic fabrics are the worst. They include acetate, acrylic, nylon, rayon, polyester, triacetate, and metallics. They may also deal a double whammy as far as skin irritation is concerned because they don't absorb perspiration.

Apparel can also give rise to allergy when nickel is involved, and zippers and other fasteners usually contain this metal. Nickel is responsible for more allergies than any other metal.

Dry cleaning processes pose another concern. They use a number of strong solvents; namely, alcohol, gasoline, kerosene, chloroform, carbon tetrachloride, perchloroethylene, benzene, acetone, naphtha, turpentine and ether. If the cleaner has stored the clothes in a plastic bag, all the worse for the allergic sensitive. These chemicals will be temporarily sealed in.

On a similar note, there are those who have developed an allergy to rubber. Items containing this substance that are worn may include belts, bras, girdles, suspenders, garter belts, gloves, boots, and the like.

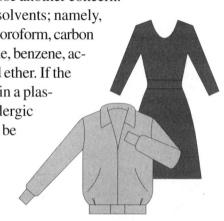

Allergies can result from exposure to chemical treatments in clothing.

Items Containing Sponge Rubber

Rubber in another form often lays in wait for its allergy victims. Sponge rubber pillows, upholstery, mattresses, seat cushions and the like throw out their share of problems. Even something as unsuspecting as rug backings, foam backed drapes, rubber-tiled floors or the rubber insulation of electric blankets are often overlooked.

Some allergy sufferers, unfortunately, have gone to the trouble of substituting sponge rubber items for bedding in which they were allergic only to become susceptible in a worse way to the fumes that emanate from the rubber. This holds especially true for electric blankets or heating pads because the transmission of the fumes into the air are intensified by high temperatures.

Those sensitive to sponge rubber can experience flushing of the face, insomnia, restlessness, depression, fatigue or night sweats.

Mattresses

Mattresses may not only contain formaldehyde, but they are required to contain flame-retardant chemicals. Pesticides, believe it or not, are also included in their manufacture.

Jewelry

Often a person's chronic skin irritation can be linked to jewelry. Nickel again comes into play if a sensitive person is wearing necklaces, bracelets or related articles that contains this metal.

And that's not all. Perspiration will dissolve nickel. This may explain why some are not bothered in winter, but are when the weather turns warmer.

In addition, symptoms can sometime persist even after suspected jewelry is long removed because nickel molecules have a propensity for attaching themselves to the cells of the skin.

Other metals can also cause allergenic problems, particularly silver and copper. And just as with nickel, the matter can be complicated by perspiration. Gold is much less implicated in allergy unless it becomes tarnished.

Air Filters

Ironically, many may depend on air filters to trap allergens, but the filters themselves may be causing problems of their own. Some may be treated with oils, adhesives, and/or plastic resins. It might also be stated that fiberglass filters can release glass fibers into the air after they have aged.

Electric Motors

Motor-driven devices such as fans, refrigerators air conditioners, electric can openers, food processors, sewing machines, and drills release some degree of ozone and oil fumes. Even this could lead to an allergy.

Heating Fuels

Natural gas, kerosene, coal, wood, or any other fuel employed for heating emits its share of gaseous or particulate matter.

The major constituents of natural gas are hydrocarbons, which are released during incomplete combustion. (No heating device, no matter how perfectly designed or maintained, is 100% efficient in burning fuel.) Furthermore, there are chemical additives present, including the one that gives the gas its familiar odor to aid in the detection of its presence for safety's sake. In other words, every time a gas heater or oven is activated, the burner may be emitting substances such as ethane, benzene, acetylene, formaldehyde, carbon monoxide, nitric oxide and nitrogen dioxide, as well as hydrogen sulfide (one of the odorants). Hydrogen sulfide alone can result in irritation to the eyes or respiratory tissue.

Even the pilot lights of heaters not in operation can affect particularly sensitive individuals. If that's not enough, even when heating appliances are shut down, minute amounts of raw fuel (some too small for even the gas company to detect) invariably escape from pipe joints and the valves themselves. Still, the story is not complete. Persons have been known to be bothered by disconnected gas appliances because their metal has the ability to absorb the vapors.

Kerosene (known to some as coal oil) can also be a serious offender. Its vapors, raw and in the burning state, can be just as harmful. If any of the oil is spilled, fumes can remain for worrisomely long periods—months or even years. Even the most ardent cleaning efforts are not completely effective.

Coal gives rise to coal dust. Even the utmost in careful handling will send a certain degree of particles aloft, not to mention the fact that it, just as any fuel, will contribute its share of pollution during the combustion process. Particularly prominent is the discharge of sulfur dioxide, an eye, skin and mucous membrane irritant, which is best known today for its connection with acid rain.

Even burning wood renders such contaminants as carbon monoxide, methane, methanol (wood alcohol), tar, sulfur dioxide, fluorene and nitrogen dioxide. But if that wood has been chemically treated, all the worse. While it's true that most of these combustible remains travel out a chimney, some amount of residue will remain inside.

Gasoline

Although gasoline burning as a fuel in internal combustion engines can be of concern for many who are allergically sensitive, the raw product deserves a billing of its own. An allergy may be initiated from the inhalation of vapors from a can of stored gasoline in a room adjacent to an attached garage. These vapors cannot only sneak in where they are not wanted through air vents, but penetrate the wall, seep through the extremities of a doorway, or escape via the attic and makes its way back into a room from the ceiling, especially in the area around light fixtures. Vapors can also escape from the filled tanks of lawn mowers, edgers, power saws, motorcycles, and the like, not to mention the family car.

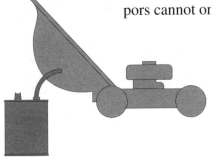

Gasoline vapors can seep into the house from storage containers and the gas tanks of power equipment and automobiles housed in attached garages.

If a susceptible one should use gasoline as a cleaning agent, the matter will be worse. He or she will be more closely exposed to it both by inhalation and contact with the skin.

Tobacco Smoke

Whether involving cigarettes, cigars, or pipes, this habit is bad enough for anyone, not only for the smoker, but for those breathing the secondhand smoke. It's health hazards have been widely publicized. But it rates a word of mention. Tobacco smoke contains, not a handful, not dozens, but in the neighborhood of an unbelievable 1500 to 3000 chemicals and other pollutants. Besides the well-known tar and nicotine, there are such harmful substances as carbon monoxide, benzene, pyrene, fluoranthene, nitrogen dioxide, formaldehyde, methane, cadmium, lead, phenols, ammonia, aluminum, sulfur, carbon disulfide, toluene, and pyridine not to mention heavy dust and other particulate matter.

As an additional slap in the face, tobacco is often treated with insecticides, as is any other crop. Even the stored leaf is vulnerable to insect attack and may be protected by fumigants. Residues will likely remain on the finished product.

On top of all that, the curing process usually requires the use of heating fuel, which can be in the form of wood, coal, coke, charcoal, oil, kerosene or liquid petroleum gas. Regardless of what kind is used, some amount of the combustible remains are absorbed by the leaf. Once the product captures a dose of it, it can never be removed— even if there is an attempt made to do so.

Even that's not all! Since tobacco is tasteless, there are many additives in the way of flavorings and sweeteners that are included in it. And they are composed of synthetic chemicals.

All of this, of course, can lead to serious illness. If burning tobacco is capable of that, it can cause allergies at the very least. In fact, the secondhand smoke broadens the chance that a child will develop an allergy or asthma if constantly exposed to it during the first 3 to 4 years of life.

Lighter Fluids

Where there's smoke (from burning tobacco, that is), there's probably lighter fluid. This is another strong chemical that, in itself, may trigger an allergy. Allergic reactions can even pop up in a family of nonsmokers if charcoal lighter fluid is used for backyard barbecues.

Plastics

This modern miracle of science also has its drawbacks. Probably taken more for granted than any other manufactered material, its wide use is virtually unlimited, being employed for such a variety of products as toys, grocery bags, laundry baskets, furniture, ball point pens, eating utensils, telephones, televisions, computers, automatic dishwashers, clothing, hand bags, costume jewelry, band-aids, lamp shades, eyeglasses, contact lenses, water beds and automobile dashboards.

Also recognized under such headings as acetate, acrylic, polyester, polyurethane, polystyrene, cellulose, nylon and vinyl, most people think of plastic as an inert material. But it is not. To some degree it outgasses because of the evaporation of resins (its chief constituent), plasticizers, stabilizers, antioxidants, solvents, colorants, and other such components.

The softer the plastic, the greater the amount of vapors escape into the air. A rain coat or shower curtain, for example, would outgas more than eyeglass frames. Also, the newer the item, the more this process takes place. A brand new beach ball would pose a much greater concern than a comb that has been around for years. In addition, heat intensifies outgassing. A heated lamp shade, therefore, is worse than a teflon pan resting in a kitchen cabinet. The phenomenon of plastic outgassing is often evident in automobiles, especially when new, which originates from the upholstery and dashboards.

One easily overlooked situation involving plastic originates from electronic items such as TVs. When hot, they give off odors, particularly from the plastic coating on the wires.

Although no allergic person is necessarily affected by every kind of plastic, many have remained fatigued and achy owing to outgassing. Chances are if one has become susceptible to general household chemicals, there will be some weakness in this direction too. One publicized account told of a woman who advanced from a status of mildly allergic to one of semi-invalid within an eight-year period in part because of her habit of wrapping all her possessions (foods, shoes, clothing, etc.) in plastic.

Paper Products

Even paper items can make a contribution to allergy. Toilet paper, tissue paper, towels, cups, plates, waxed paper, shelf paper and even grocery sacks contain formaldehyde, which is included in the manufacturing process because it augments the wet strength of the product. Shelf paper may even contain insecticide! In the case of scented and tinted items, such as toilet and tissue paper, other chemicals are added as well. In addition, some white paper is bleached with chlorine.

Office Supplies and Equipment

Office supplies at work or at home can be causing some allergy victims grief. Rubber cement and the ink from felt-tipped pens are especially noteworthy. Problems can also rise from photocopying equipment and laser printers. They release a measure of ozone and the vapors from the inks used find their way into the air, when the devices are in operation.

Construction Materials

One can also be affected by materials used in carpentry. On the list: particle board, insulating materials, fiberglass, vinyl, wallpaper and carpeting. Many of them contain formaldehyde as well as toluene and other such substances.

Carpets can be particularly troublesome because they can harbor mold and other particulate matter when they become damp. As it is, carpets and rugs accumulate a host of contaminants over time from shoes, pets and just what falls from the air. According to one study, in fact, carpeting was found to collect a hundred times the rate of allergens as that of bare floors. And the thick-pile variety, of course, is worse than the low-pile. In addition, carpets are impregnated with dirt-repellent coatings, mothproofing, fungicides, fire retardants and dyes. The carpet itself can eventually become a problem due to normal wear and tear, which causes microscopic bits of material to break off and be lifted into the air by foot traffic, where they are circulated in heating and air conditioning systems. This can prove doubly bad in winter when they are heated because that changes their chemistry. Carpeting made from natural fibers is bad enough, but those containing synthetic fibers are capable of producing over a hundred different compounds, including sulfuric acid and hydrogen cyanide.

Wallpaper, too, poses more problems than meet the eye. To begin with, wallpaper paste usually contains insecticides and fungicides. These chemicals penetrate the paper and are sometimes even incorporated in the paper itself. Wallpapers made from fabric present another problem. The surface often breaks down into cellulose dust. Bits of fiberglass can flake off of fiberglass wallpaper and vinyl wallpaper will release vinyl chloride vapors. Ink and paints used for printed designs outgas their chemical content as well.

Solder

When heat is applied to it, solder releases vapors into the air. One of these substances is lead, as solder is composed of 60% of this metal.

Condoms

This contraceptive can also become an allergen. It may be the rubber itself or a powder or lubricant it bears. Swelling and rashes anywhere in the genital region can result in the man or his partner, or even both. Some brands may be tolerated while others are not.

Toys

Stuffed toys can be a problem for children for the same reason as stuffed furniture, pillows and other such items can for anyone. And just think of how many toys are made from plastic that releases its vapors into the air.

Scented Candles

Many have been cautioned about "burning the candle at both ends," but burning it at just one end may be bad enough. Scented candles that see the end of a lighted match may smell delightful, but they can burden the air with substances that are troublesome for the chemically sensitive. Even the unscented variety releases a certain amount of combustibles into the air.

Mustaches and Beards

Do you believe you could be allergic to yourself? Technically, there is no truth to this, but your facial hair might be harboring allergens that may have accumulated there throughout the day. According to Springfield, Virginia allergist Patricia McNally, "Men who suffer from pollen allergies and who sport a mustache are at a much higher risk for developing symptoms than men without mustaches." And, of course, that would put beards not too far behind.

Water Beds

Water beds could be creating problems for many. Although they may be a better choice than a mattress for those allergic to airborne particles such as dust mites, they won't help those who react to plastic outgassing. What makes them particularly noteworthy is the fact that one sleeps on them for hours each night, and thereby receives lengthy periods of exposure. To make matters worse, the heat from the sleeper's body will increase the amount of plastic outgassing. And if they should spring a leak, that would be an open invitation for mold proliferation.

Table 21

Other Items that can Trigger Allergies	
Air filters	Office supplies and equipment
Clothing	Paper products
Condoms	Plastics
Construction materials	Rubber
Electric motors	Solder
Gasoline	Toys
Heating fuels	Tobacco smoke
Jewelry	Water beds
Lighter fluids	

Activities that can Generate Particulate Matter

Filing, sanding, planing and drilling cause the particulate count of the surrounding air to zoom upward. Tiny bits of wood, metal, plastic or other material can be readily breathed. Even writing on a blackboard can release chalk dust. A high enough concentration of any particulate matter will reduce lung function and increase the load on the heart, and even small amounts can cause an allergy.

That covers the allergens. Now let's get down to the business of solving allergenic problems.

Part 3:
Solutions

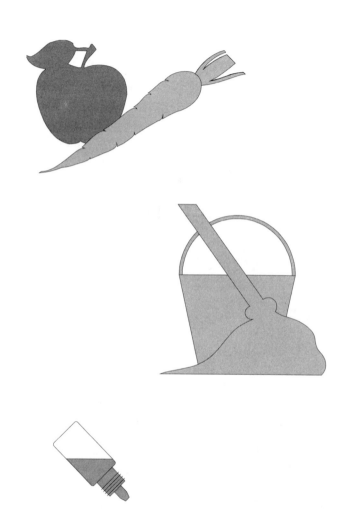

Chapter 12
Finding the Answer to Your Allergy Problem

As you can see, unearthing answers to allergy problems is often a difficult chore. Fortunately, it doesn't always have to be. In any case, since you have read this far you may have already diagnosed your allergy and, hopefully have a much better idea about what you can do. In fact, by this time you might have solved your dilemma. If not, you will hopefully turn up the solution in the pages that follow.

First, let's lay the groundwork. Generally, in order to find relief from allergic symptoms, one must consider the following:

• Avoidance

• Elimination

• Reduction

• Substitution

• Improved diet

If, for instance, you are allergic to pollen, your first step is to avoid it as much as possible. Should you discover a susceptibility to face creams, you eliminate them. If you have an allergy to dust mites, you reduce the content of them as much as you can. If your problem lies with aspirin, you search for an aspirin-free medication that will do the job. In the event you react adversely to additives in processed foods, you concentrate on enriching your diet with plenty of fresh foods.

As we've seen, however, there are other factors to consider even after the diagnosis of an allergy and the isolation of its cause. An allergen cannot always be avoided. It may be difficult to eliminate because there are many ingredients common to different products. There may be accidental contamination from one substance to that of another. Then there is the possibility of multiple allergies.

With the application of common sense and a little detective work, however, these challenges can often be overcome. Let's explore the positive steps that can be instituted for a more allergy-free life.

Chapter 13
Getting Tough with Airborne Allergens

The first move to make when an allergy to airborne matter is involved is to eliminate as much of it as is practical from your life. You can't do anything about the out-of-doors, but you can control what's inside. This can be accomplished in several ways. You can:

- Clean thoroughly
- Filter it more efficiently
- Control humidity

Vacuuming

The most common way to remove dust and other particulate matter is to vacuum it up. You can't get it all, of course, but you can improve the situation. Unfortunately, while conventional vacuum cleaners make the carpets look good, they are not very efficient at trapping the smaller bits of dust and debris, those that can more easily enter the respiratory system of a sensitive person. They are utterly sucked up and blown back out through the porous bag (the only means of exhaust the device possesses) to be redistributed into the air.

The only line of defense in this case is to wear a filter mask while cleaning. The cotton surgical kind will often suffice, the best choice of

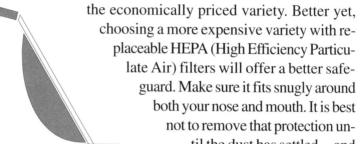

the economically priced variety. Better yet, choosing a more expensive variety with replaceable HEPA (High Efficiency Particulate Air) filters will offer a better safeguard. Make sure it fits snugly around both your nose and mouth. It is best not to remove that protection until the dust has settled—and that may be as much as an hour. It is also highly advisable to empty the vacuum cleaner bag out-of-doors to avoid the reintroduction of matter into the indoor environment. Additionally, it is

Conventional vacuum cleaners don't remove the smaller particles, those that create many allegies. Vacuuming devices with replaceable HEPA filers will offer a better safeguard.

better to replace the bag when only half full, to clean the area around the bag with a moist cloth before installing a fresh bag, and to run the machine for at least 30 seconds before returning it to the house so any loose dust that remains will be expelled.

Fortunately, there are alternatives. Accessory filters are available that can be added to some conventional vacuum cleaners (the canister type; *e. g.*, the kind employing a hard outer shell), thereby reducing the number of particles they emit.

Another option is to invest in a more efficient vacuuming device. There are a number of other varieties on the market that use a filter that is capable of removing much smaller particles.

There is also a kind of portable vacuuming unit that depends on a basin of water to trap the dirt. It is generally known as a water-trap vacuum cleaner. All water-soluble material that is pulled in is absorbed by the swirling liquid. The dirty water can be emptied after cleaning is complete with no fear of recontaminating the air.

Sweeping Vs. Mopping

While sweeping may seem like a good habit, it can stir up a lot of tiny debris. In addition, a certain amount of these particles remain on the broom itself, some to be released by air currents whenever a closet door is opened, for instance, or perhaps liberated the next time one puts the broom into action.

Mopping is a better choice for keeping down the airborne count. Most of the dust and dirt picked up by the mop is trapped by the moistening agent applied to the strands. When the mop is rinsed, the contaminants are washed away. If you happen to be chemically sensitive, don't use a strong cleaner, merely moisten the mop with water.

In short, the best rule is "sweep sparingly, mop frequently."

Overlooked Items that Accumulate Dust

There are a number of areas often overlooked that harbor dust. Some examples: refrigerator tops, ceiling light fixtures, the ornate carvings of the more intricate varieties of furniture, upper shelves and closets. Even the top portion of ceiling fans require attention, especially if they have been idle for a while.

Exhaust fans are often passed over. They must be cleaned occasionally or they cannot be relied upon to adequately remove dusty air. The cover plate can be removed and placed in hot soapy water. While it is soaking in the sink, wipe out the exhaust opening, preferably with an environmentally friendly cleaner such as a mixture of borax and water. The motor unit can also be removed and brushed off. (Don't expose it to water, however, as this could prove harmful to the mechanism.)

If you have electric baseboard heaters, they need to be cleaned too, as they have a tendency to collect a lot of dust, as do wall radiators. You can gain access to the dirt by removing the protective cover.

Table 22

Overlooked Items that Accumulate Dust	
Baseboard heaters	Exhaust fans
Ceiling fans	Refrigerator tops
Ceiling light fixtures	Upper shelves
Closets	Wall radiators

Making Dusting Matters Easier

Don't make it hard on yourself. Say good-bye to "dust catchers." Any knickknacks or odd-shaped items difficult to dust around are fair game. This includes such articles as old books and magazines. Even bed canopies count, as they are big dust catchers over time. It never costs anything to discard and there are a number of things one can always find to part with.

Don't crowd closets with too many possessions. A surprising amount of dust can find its way inside even when the doors have been tightly shut. Also consider the use of a wire shoe rack. When cleaning closet floors, it can be much more quickly removed than individual pairs of shoes.

Other useful tips: Try replacing hanging light fixtures—especially chandeliers—with recessed lighting. Also, cover baseboard heaters and wall radiators in the summer time.

In extreme cases, it may become necessary to eliminate upholstery, draperies, venetian blinds and carpeting. Unstuffed furniture, washable cotton curtains (recommended as a good substitute for heavy draperies by most allergists), window shades or shutters, and hard wood flooring receive a green light. Other environmentally friendly materials include terrazzo, ceramic tile, formica, glass, marble, porcelain, stone and metals.

If a child's room is involved, it would be a good idea to keep a minimum amount of toys in the room, and the ones that remain should be of the washable variety. No stuffed toys should be included. All toys should be kept in a box with a lid, not resting on open shelves. Box springs and mattresses should be covered in a dust-proof casing—and nothing should ever be stored under the bed. Bunk beds should also be avoided.

Clothing in closets should be hung and sealed in garment bags. Of course, make sure the attire, as well as bedspreads, covers, sheets, and curtains are washed regularly and dried thoroughly. When washing bedding, make sure the temperature of the water exceeds 130° Fahrenheit. Dust mites cannot live at this temperature. For good measure, set your automatic drier to the hottest possible setting.

Giving Dust Mites the Deep Freeze

While dust mites cannot live beyond 130° Fahrenheit, they also have an equal problem with cold temperatures, and you can take advantage of this. Any stuffed toys your children consider absolutely indispensable that you can't throw in the washer can be placed in the freezer for an hour every week. This won't remove the mites, but it will kill them, halting their reproduction.

Note: Water beds, although not recommended for those sensitive to plastic, are a reasonable alternative to conventional beds for holding down particulate matter, as there is no padding to collect dust or to furnish a campsite for dust mites. But keep an eye out for any leaks, which will invite the growth of mold.

If you do possess carpeting in any part of your place of residence, or stuffed furniture, they should be steam-cleaned at least every few years. This especially holds true for the bedroom, the place where you spend 8 hours or so every night.

Better yet, it is probably best to follow the advice of Diana Marquardt, chief of the allergy-immunology department at the University of California, San Diego, Medical Center, who in regard to bedrooms, suggests, "You should only have items in the room that you can pick up and wash in hot water—including upholstery, curtains and rugs—and you should wash these materials every week, at best."

Air Filtration

Air purifiers can also help the cause. The small table models found in department stores and drug stores are the most economical way to go. They may remove enough airborne matter to benefit some of the less susceptible.

However, they will not suffice for serious situations. For a more thorough job, there are purifiers that use HEPA filters.

A HEPA filter is made from extremely thin glass fibers pressed into a pleated paper. The HEPA filter is customarily piggybacked with two other kinds of filters: a pre-filter for capturing larger particles (to protect the HEPA filter from becoming clogged) and an activated charcoal filter for absorbing certain odors. Purifiers using HEPA filters are capable of removing the vast majority of the foreign matter in the air. In fact, they meet rigid industrial standards and are utilized in such places as electronic chip manufactering facilities and operating rooms.

Other portable devices for cleaning the air come in the form of electronic (or electrostatic) air cleaners. These portable units charge particles electronically and pull them out of the air, where they are deposited on a special plate. They are not, however, as efficient as HEPA filters and their efficiency tends to drop over time. In addition, they produce a small measure of ozone. Ozone in small concentrations may not pose any problems, but it can induce eye irritation and headaches in some. If you know you are sensitive to ozone, you will have to explore one of the other alternatives.

A similar kind of portable electronic air cleaner is a negative-ion generator. It generates negatively charged ions that intercept particles and pull them back to a filter in the unit. The generator, however, also emits ozone.

There are also electrostatic filters designed for central air systems, but they too release ozone. Much more efficient passive filters intended to replace the conventional kind are also available for this application.

Another idea is to install charcoal filter pads to each of the room vents of central air systems. In addition, it is good policy to have the air ducts professionally cleaned every few years. They can easily remain one of the most contaminated places in the house because they are so inaccessible for cleaning and such as large percentage of the matter in the air circulates through them.

Controlling Humidity

In any case, no matter how you go about otherwise reducing the airborne allergen count, it is advisable to keep the humidity at a low enough level. Not only does this offer maximum comfort to the body, but it discourages the proliferation of bacteria, mold and dust mites. Besides, dust has a habit of clinging to moisture in the air. If your home is not equipped with a dehumidifier (either as part of the central air system or as a portable unit), it would be wise to invest in one if high humidity is a problem, such as it is in coastal regions or areas near lakes.

The kitchen and bathroom are the most vulnerable places in the home, because that is where most of the moisture exists. Pay attention to vegetable bins, drip trays, and the rubber gaskets on the doors of refrigerator and freezer. Check for leaking sink pipes, drippy faucets and sluggish drains. Make any necessary repairs to plumbing and clean out the drains. Also examine the bottom of cold-water pipes. Baths, showers, and general washing contributes to mold growth. Use a squeegee on glass shower doors after bathing or showering. Wipe the surfaces of bathtubs and shower stalls with a towel after each use. Wash and dry bath mats regularly. Spread out used towels and stretch out shower curtains. As it is, there is a standing bowl of water constantly present in the toilet, so keep the rear base of toilets and the floor immediately surrounding them clean and dry. Check tile grouting, another potential trouble spot. Clean or re-grout where necessary. Make any neccessary repairs to plumbing and clean out the drains.

If you have a basement, you must be responsive to conditions there also. Although condensation is enough of a problem, it is not the only contributor to moisture there. Any water that accumulates in the ground around the house will press against basement walls, especially near the bottom where pressure is at its highest, and eventually work its way in through cracks, gaps and joints.

Any imperfections should be patched to keep moisture outside. A good compound to employ is hydraulic cement, a quick-setting substance sold at paint and hardware stores, which expands upon contact with water. It can even be used while water is seeping through.

To confirm the origin of a moisture problem, tightly tape a piece of aluminum foil to the basement wall when it is dry. When dampness recurs, if the side of the foil facing you is wet, the problem is condensation. But if the side that has been contacting the wall is moist, water is penetrating the wall from the outside.

Also inspect other areas in and around the house where unanticipated moisture could accumulate. Check window-mounted air conditioners for standing water and supply adequate drainage if needed. Make sure the insulation surrounding central air vents is intact. If any of it has come off, moisture can build up inside them. Check rainspouts to make certain an excess amount of water isn't building up too closely to the foundation. If a problem of this nature exists, reroute the flow of water by using an extension or installing concrete troughs. And don't hold still for a leaky roof.

It's also a good idea to check outdoor shrubbery. Hedges planted too close to outside walls can impede airflow and reduce evaporation in the lower extremities of the house. This holds especially true for walls that don't receive much sunlight. Trim back or remove any plants that are suspect. This has an added advantage in that any pollen-producing plant growth that might be contributing to hay fever will be gone.

During the day, keep drapes open so that condensed air won't form on the windows. Another way to minimize the creation and collection of moisture is to install double windows.

Make sure your home is adequately insulated. Poorly insulated structure will admit warm, moist air into the wall cavities where it will promote not only fungal growth, but condensation damage. Even the air leaking through an inadequately sealed electrical outlet during the winter months will pull in more moisture than what can defuse through 1,000 square feet of a typical plaster wall.

This warning, however: If the humidity level gets too low, it cannot only play its part in encouraging dust to become airborne, but it will create a drying effect upon the protective linings of the nose, throat and lungs.

At any rate, a relative humidity level in the range of 40% to 60% is recommended by the experts. Hygrometers, devices that measure this condition, are inexpensive and relatively available.

Another tip: Maintain a lower-than-average temperature. While this is no substitute for cleaning, it will at least help somewhat in keeping down the airborne particulate count.

Avoiding Outside Particulate Matter

In regard to the out-of-doors, you may have to avoid it whenever practical, when conditions are less than ideal. A lot of particulate debris can be stirred up on windy days, and of course dust storms make the worst possible scenario. The best times to be outside under normal conditions, if you have a choice, is during the morning hours, before the hustle and bustle of daily activity begins, or just after a rain shower because precipitation washes particles out of the air. If pollen is your concern, you'll have to avoid the early mornings as well as late evenings whenever possible because pollen levels are generally highest at those times. Pollen is less troublesome on cool, cloudy, windless days. Conditions are also more favorable during times of high humidity because pollen is not released then.

When working outside, those who are particularly sensitive to pollen or mold should wear a face mask. The eyes should also be protected with goggles. Lawn mowing, raking leaves, even gardening will stir up the grass and soil, releasing a large dose of both of these allergens. Also, in regard to mold, Peter J. Casano, an allergy specialist and otolaryngologist in Jackson, Mississippi, states, "You should also watch out for especially damp areas when hiking or camping.

Dark areas with rotting logs or stagnant water can also be home to a number of different types of mold, so don't set up camp next to a pond."

Reducing Gaseous Matter

Contaminants in the form of gas must be handled differently. Gases exist on a molecular level and cannot be screened by conventional mechanical filtration. They are best avoided by remaining indoors as much as possible whenever there is a notable pollution problem in the outside air, and don't open windows or doors unnecessarily during those times. Also, don't generate your own pollution inside by using strong chemicals. Under normal conditions, if you have a choice, pick times to go outside when there is no rush hour traffic. The early morning hours are better than those later in the day, because the air will be freer from gaseous pollutants. It's also a good idea to keep an eye on wind direction. This is important whenever you are situated downwind from a busy highway or a factory.

If your problem is associated with natural gas, you have a lot of options. You can install an exhaust fan above your kitchen range if you don't already have one. This may reduce emissions as much as 50%. Cooking more slowly also helps. The reduced temperatures will lessen the rate of contamination as well as the chance of boil-overs, which deposits food residue on burners, thereby creating an additional brand of pollution. Low-temperature cooking has another advantage. Fats that are subjected to high temperatures can affect some chemically sensitive people. Also consider cooking food as briefly as possible. This has another advantage too: More of the nourishing substances will be retained. Using hot

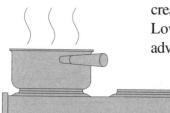

Gaseous contaminants can be reduced by cooking more slowly and for shorter periods of time.

plates and steamers whenever appropriate also helps limit natural gas emissions.

As for heating the house with a gas-fired central air system, the best one can do is keep the thermostat on the lowest practical setting so the heater will shut off more often. Of course, you should keep your heater, as well as any gas stoves, well maintained. The burning efficiency of neglected gas equipment can be cut to as much as half of what it is when new. And that puts more contaminants in the air.

You may be so sensitive that you are forced to give up gas heating all together. A heat pump system or electric baseboard heaters are better choices. You might also consider supplementary solar heat. As for portable devices, stick with fan-forced or radiant electric heaters.

If you suspect you are experiencing grief from gaseous matter, you may have to start removing certain home furnishings, such as upholstery (including synthetic and tanned leather headboards), mattresses, bedding covers and drapes, because they are treated with a number of chemicals. And don't forget about plastic materials. Substitute furniture with little or no padding. Untreated wood furnishings are a good choice. You might even try items made of wicker, wrought iron or steel with a baked enamel finish. Untreated cotton mattresses, covers and drapes are also better choices.

And here's something you may not have considered: using house plants to filter the air. That's right! Air contamination research for NASA has proven it. Although they cannot be depended upon heavily, spider plants are capable of removing small amounts of formaldehyde from the air. Golden pothos, philodendrons and snake plants will help in this regard too. In addition, one can combat benzene to some extent by keeping chrysanthemums and gerbera daises. For air purification in general, try aloe and banana trees, arneca palm, arrowhead vine, Boston fern, Chinese evergreen, dracaena, dwarf date palm, English ivy, mother-in-law's tongue, peace lily and reed palm. These plants also release a substance that reduces airborne concentrations of mold spores and bacteria. Just 1 or 2 plants are all that is required for every 100 square feet. So unless you are extremely sensitive to mold, this may be the way to go. Let mother nature do its share of the air filtering.

What About the Car?

When traveling in your car, keep rear windows closed. A fact unrecognized by many is that passengers riding in back seats with windows open—even a crack—are exposed to a dose of their own automobile's exhaust fumes because the vehicle's motion creates a vacuum behind itself which will capture some of the contaminants and suck them inside. This suggests that numerous cases of car sickness may really be nothing more than a set of symptoms that have been brought on by this phenomena.

Even front windows, to some measure, can pose the same problem. For this reason, it is better to keep all windows closed while driving. As it is, a certain amount of chemical contaminants will seep inside anyway.

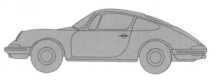

Keep windows closed while driving. Even while in motion, a motor vehicle will capture some of its own exhaust fumes and suck them inside.

Don't use any outside air intakes, often labeled "fresh air" or "mix" on the dash, because it will do nothing more than bring in "fresh" air from the road, containing not only exhaust fumes, but sometimes a host of other unexpected surprises such as emanations from freshly tarred streets, factories, sewers, or even pesticide sprayings, as well as fumes from the engine. The same thing applies to the heater because it also will pull in a certain degree of these contaminants. The best policy is to dress adequately, and limit the use of the heater. In summer, it is often difficult to escape running the air conditioner, but many factory-installed units will invite in a certain percentage of outside air. If this is so in your case, consider having one of the recirculating variety installed.

No matter what kind of air conditioner you have, it is better to use it than to open windows. If you keep it on maximum cool, the increased pressure from it helps to prevent fumes from entering. This holds an added advantage because a car with a cooler interior will outgas less. And do not neglect the air conditioner filter. It should be replaced periodically. And while you're at it, have the vents cleaned.

Whenever you have control over the time you drive, do it in the mornings, particularly before rush hour when the air is fresher or at least after the traffic has subsided. This especially holds true in the summertime when the hot afternoon air is usually packed with a higher measure of pollution.

To help deter contaminants from finding their way inside, use judgment in how you drive by simple observation. Be alert to which way the wind is blowing by watching which direction the smoke from factories, diesel trucks or the like is moving, or perhaps by taking note of tree movement. Adjust your driving accordingly by remaining on the desirable side of vehicles when possible. Also, stay a reasonable distance behind the vehicle ahead of you, especially if it's a bus or a truck. Avoid tunnels, which are notorious for trapping fumes. Stick to the side roads whenever practical. And never idle your car unnecessarily.

Of course, vehicles in disrepair, such as those with defective mufflers or ones that are poorly tuned, must be attended to. As might be expected, the more smoke that is visible from an exhaust system, the more inefficient the engine is operating and, therefore, the more combustibles there are released into the air.

It's also wise to check the general integrity of your automobile. Unexpected problems may crop up if there is a way for contaminants to get inside easily. To give you an idea of what can happen, one young man became plagued with exhaustion, dizziness, depression and a number of other symptoms when a crack in the rubber at the base of the floor-mounted stick shift of his sports car allowed vapors from the heated up engine to seep inside the snug, 2-seat compartment.

Another thing to remember, and it goes without saying, when filling the tank of your vehicle, avoid breathing the gasoline fumes emitted from the pump.

What You Can Do at Work?

You may not have total control at your workplace, but here are some basic suggestions for reducing the load of contaminants upon you, if and when the opportunity avails itself. Avoid areas where airborne allergens are generated or are likely to linger. Try to reduce the pollutants you breath by opening a window if possible. Leave the building as often as you are permitted and take advantage of the fresh air outside, unless you are situated in the heart of an industrial area or someplace else where heavy pollution exists. Consider using an air purifier. Never neglect to wear protective gear whenever the job calls for it. Avoid the inhalation of strong vapors from chemical products such as rubber cement and felt-tip markers. Substitute a less odorous office supplies such as glue and ball-point pens when applicable. Also shy away from operating laser printers or photocopy machines whenever possible. And, above all, run from cigarette smoke.

Table 23

Taking Precautions at Work

- Avoid areas where airborne allergens are generated or are likely to linger.
- Open window if possible.
- Leave the building as often as you are permitted.
- Use an air purifier.
- Wear protective gear whenever the job calls for it.
- Avoid the inhalation of strong vapors from chemical products.
- Substitute less odorous office supplies when applicable.
- Avoid inhaling fumes from operating laser printers or photocopy machines.
- Avoid tobacco smoke.

Bear in mind that your symptoms may not subside immediately after your shift ends. They may linger all weekend or throughout your days off. Just because you don't start feeling better as soon as you leave the office does not necessarily mean you don't have an allergy produced from there. If you are not certain, institute as many of the measures presented above as you can.

Chapter 14
A Diet to Discourage Allergy

In order to be victorious over food allergies, you must first be fully aware of everything you are eating. Avoid the food in which you suspect you have a sensitivity for 4 to 6 weeks. This strategy, known as an elimination diet, will purge your system of all traces of the food and rest your body from its effects. Take note of how you feel during that period. You may feel worse rather than better for the first 4 or 5 days because you have withdrawn something your body has been receiving regularly. But stick with it. If your symptoms eventually disappear, you have probably isolated the allergen. Then try the food again to make sure. In fact, unless you are highly sensitive, feel free to splurge on it for good measure. If symptoms reappear, you have your answer.

Don't make a hasty deduction, though. A delayed reaction could occur that might not surface for 18 hours or more after ingestion of the suspected food. Also note that further experimentation with the culprit may reveal a surprise. You might discover you can tolerate small amounts of it with no ill effects.

In the case of multiple food allergies, you will have to test yourself by removing other edibles from your diet. Concentrate on one at a time. During this period you should skirt around commercially processed foods, as they can complicate matters. You may, for instance, have an allergy to eggs, but it won't do you much good to stop eating omelets for breakfast, and continue indulging in cake for desserts, which contain eggs as part of their recipe. Nor will it help if you give up corn and continue drinking canned fruit juices that contain corn syrup. For this same reason, you should avoid eating out, unless you are sure of all the contents of the foods being served.

Instead, stick to fresh produce as much as you can. This action alone may alleviate your symptoms. These nutritious foods are packed with vitamins, minerals, and other essential substances. And unknown to many, vegetables contain a significant amount of protein when enough of them are eaten. Including organically grown items in your diet is all the better. You may discover your allergic reactions have been triggered by lingering residues of a pesticide.

You might have to maintain a "food diary" if matters become difficult for you. It should include a list of all foods consumed, as well as their quantity, and the time they were eaten, along with any symptoms that occur and the time in which they are noticed. Remember to include all the ingredients of any dishes that you prepare. And don't leave chewing gum off the list. Although it is not swallowed, the contents of the gum is ingested via the saliva.

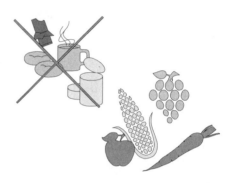

Forsaking processed foods for fresh produce is an excellent step toward solving food allergy problems.

It is wise to begin the diary before any alterations are made to your diet and continue it for a short time after you have completed your tests. Don't begin if you are sick. Wait until the illness has passed. The less matters there are to complicate the results, the better. Don't attempt an elimination diet if you have experienced severe reactions to foods.

As stated above, things will go much better if you desist from all processed foods. Otherwise, you will have to record in your diary every ingredient on every can and package label to get accurate results from your diet. One miss and a problematic additive or soy derivative may slip past you.

This will not go without effort, but the rewards can be great.

The Rotation Diet

Some have embarked upon a rotation diet in an attempt to control food sensitivities, and it deserves a word here. Menus are arranged so that biologically related foods are consumed on the same day and foods from that same family are not reintroduced for at least 4 days, the maximum interval it requires for all traces of a food to exit the body. For instance, on the first day, one might concentrate on the potato family by eating potatoes, tomatoes, eggplant and peppers—then the next day switching to the mustard family, which includes broccoli, Brussels sprouts, cabbage, cauliflower, collards, horseradish, kale, radishes, turnips and watercress. The pattern continues the next day, and so on. Anything, then, in the potato family could not be consumed again before the 4-day period has elapsed.

This kind of diet, however, is considered controversial by most experts because research has established that having a reaction to one food does not neccesarily mean one will be affected by others in the same group. Furthermore, extended use of this kind of diet could lead to malnutrition because balanced meals are not being consumed.

Deciphering Labels

You will probably find it difficult to give up all processed foods during an elimination diet. At the least, you will be reintroducing some, if not all, of these foods into your diet eventually. In any case, it will be helpful to familiarize yourself with how to use labels to recognize "hidden allergens" in products.

Let's take a look at the basic foods that are most commonly linked to allergies, which are often utilized as ingredients in processed products under unfamiliar names.

The Many Names of Corn

Corn may be present in any products bearing on its label terms such as "baking powder," "citric acid," "dextrose," or "food starch." See table 24 for a more comprehensive list.

Table 24

Product Label Terms Indicating the Presence of Corn

Baking powder	Maize
Caramel	Malt
Citric acid	Malt extract
Dextrates	Malt syrup
Dextrin	Maltodextrin
Dextrose	Modified food starch
Food starch	Monosodium glutamate (MSG)
Fructose	Starch
Golden syrup	Syrup
Grits	Treacle vanilla extract
Hominy	Vegetable gum
Invert sugar	Vegetable oil
Invert syrup	Vegetable starch
Lactic acid	Xanthan gum

Hidden Egg Protein

Egg protein may be incorporated into products labeled with terms such as "albumin," "binder", "coagulant," "emulsifier," "globulin," "lecithin" or "silici albuminate." The general terms such as "binder," "coagulant" and "emulsifier" merely describe the function that the egg performs. The lecithin used in the majority of manufactured food products is obtained from soy, but sometimes it may be from that of the egg instead. The term "ovo," derived from the Latin word for egg, is also a tip-off of its presence. It is often used as part of a word describing the contents of a product. "Ovomuccoid" and "ovovitellin" are examples. A more comprehensive list is included in table 25.

Unfortunately, the presence of egg is not always acknowledged on labels, as when egg whites are used to give certain baked goods such as pie crusts or bagels their shiny appearance.

Table 25

Product Label Terms Indicating the Presence of Egg Protein

Albumin	Lysozyme
Avidin	Ovalbumin
Binder	Ovamucin
Coagulant	Ovomucin
Conalbumin	Ovomucoid
Emulsifier	Ovotransferrin
Globulin	Ovovitellin
Lecithin	Phosvitin
Lipovitelin	Silici albuminate
Livetin	Vitellin

Products Containing Milk

Milk or milk derivatives can be identified in foodstuffs whose label includes such terms as: "butter," "caramel," "cheese", "cream," "half-and-half," "Kosher symbol 'D' or 'DE'," "lactose," "natural flavoring," "nougat," or "sherbet." The term "no milk fat" must also be included here. The fact that a product doesn't contain any milk fat does not mean that it's completely milk-free. See table 26 for a more comprehensive list.

Don't be put off by terms that contain the word "milk" when it describes a plant source. "Soy milk" and "rice milk" are good examples. Likewise, do not fear the terms "lactylate," "lactate" and "lactic acid." These substances don't contain milk.

Table 26

Product Label Terms Indicating the Presence of Milk or Milk Derivatives	
Butter	Kefir
Caramel	Kosher symbol "D" or "DE"
Casein	Lactalbumin
Caseinate	Lactoglobulin
Cheese	Lactose
Cream	Natural flavoring
Curd	Nougat
Dairy	Quark
Feta	Rennet casein
Ghee	Ricotta
Half-and-half	Sherbet
High-protein flavor	Whey
High-protein flour	Yogurt

The Many Faces of Wheat

Wheat may have a presence in food items labeled with such terms as "bran," "cereal extract," "crackers and cracker meal," "dextrin," "flour," "hydrolyzed vegetable protein," "modified food starch" or "stabilizers." See table 27 for a more comprehensive list.

Note: Despite its name, buckwheat is in an entirely different food family from wheat, and in its pure form is a wheat-free, as well as gluten-free seed. However, if it is included as an ingredient in a product label as "buckwheat flour" it might contain both buckwheat and wheat flours.

Table 27

Product Label Terms Indicating the Presence of Wheat	
Bran	Hydrolyzed vegetable protein
Bulgur	Kamut
Cereal extract	Maltodextrin
Couscous	Matzoh
Crackers and cracker meal	Modified food starch
Dextrin	Seasoning
Durum	Seitan
Farina	Semolina
Flour	Spelt
Glutin	Stabilizers
Graham	Surimi
Hydrolyzed plant protein	Triticale

The Presence of Nuts

Peanuts may be included in products whose terms on its label are marked with: "Asian dressing," "Asian sauce," "flavoring," "loratamine" or "mandalona." The term "arachis oil" must also be mentioned, which is actually peanut oil. Also, not only do Asian foods often contain peanuts or are contaminated with them during preparation, but so are African and Hispanic foods. Check the nationality before purchase.

Tree nuts can be found in foods whose label includes the words: "gianduja," "marzipan," "nougat," "pesto" or "pralines."

Table 28

Product Label Terms Indicating the Presence of Peanuts

Arachis oil	Flavoring
Asian dressing	Loratamine
Asian sauce	Mandalona

Table 29

Product Label Terms Indicating the Presence of Tree Nuts

Gianduja	Pesto
Marzipan	Pralines
Nougat	

Terms For Soy

Terms that sometimes or always indicate the presence of soy include "carob," "lecithin" "starch" and "hydrogentated vegetable protein" (HVP), not to mention "MSG." Just as with the egg, soy may be listed on the label according to how it is used. Often, soy serves as an emulsifier, stabilizer or thickener, for example. Check table 30 for a more comprehensive list.

Table 30

Product Label Terms that Indicate the Presence of Soy
Bulking agent
Carob
Emulsifier
Guar gum
Gum arabic
Hydrogentated vegetable protein (HVP)
Lecithin
Miso
Monosodium glutamate (MSG)
Protein
Protein extender
Shoyu
Stabilizer
Starch
Tamari
Tempeh
Textured vegetable protein (TVP)
Thickener
Tofu
Vegetable broth
Vegetable gum
Vegetable oil
Vegetable starch
Vitamin E

Where Yeast Can be Found

Yeast is contained in anything employing the term "hydrolyzed vegetable protein." Products including the word "malt" on the label indicate a secondary source of yeast. Other label terms indicating the presence of yeast in products are "au gratin," "breaded," "enriched flour," "enzymes," "flavoring," "mushroom," "sour" and "vinegar." This also includes the potential presence of mold.

Table 31

Label Terms that may or do Contain Yeast
au gratin
Breaded
Enriched flour
Enzymes
Flavoring
Hydrolyzed vegetable protein
Malt
Mushroom
Sour
Vinegar

If you rely upon packaged foods at all, examine labels carefully. The less ingredients named, the better. Lean heavily toward quick-frozen items, which don't contain chemical preservatives.

Subsitutions

Don't be discouraged when you must give up a certain food. There are numerous appealing substitutions that can be made, which taste good and are nourishing.

Alternatives for Corn

If corn is the problem, there are other grains that can be served, such as rice or oatmeal. For recipes that require a thickener and call for cornstarch, try potato starch instead. Tapioca starch or arrowroot can also used. Corn meal can be replaced with soy flour, potato meal or millet. In lieu of corn syrup, you might want to try maple syrup, brown rice syrup, molasses or even concentrated fruit juice, even though they may alter the color or flavor of the finished dish. Corn tortillas can be swapped for the flour based kind. Try potato or rice chips instead of corn chips, or popped rice instead of popcorn.

Equitable Trade-Offs for Eggs

If eggs are at the heart of your allergy, try avocados as a substitute. They possess a similar texture to boiled eggs and contain a large amount of protein. In recipes, eggs can easily be replaced by an equal amount of water or wet foods. It may be in the form of applesauce, fruit juice or even mashed bananas, not to mention water.

Baking powder works well for purposes of leavening. Baking soda can also be used for this purpose, but a sour substance such as lemon juice or vinegar must be added to it for the leavening process to take place. Beware of commercial egg substitutes. Some brands actually contain egg whites!

Milk Replacements

Should milk be your culprit, there are numerous other beverages from which to choose. For cooking, you can substitute water or any vegetable juice in recipes calling for milk. In addition, soy milk is an excellent trade-off for cow's milk. Soy contains all the essential amino acids necessary to make a complete protein just as animal milk, as well as 30 times the iron. At the same time, soy milk contains no cholesterol or lactose.

You can even fashion a light cream from nuts, believe it or not, for cooking purposes. Provided you don't have a nut allergy, take a half cup of almonds, pine nuts or filberts. Cover in water and soak overnight. Drain water the next day. Place them in a blender with enough water to cover them again, then mix into a cream. Add water if necessary to achieve the desired consistency. This should make about 1 quart.

There are dairy-free substitutes on the market for milk, as well as butter and cheese, which you may prefer instead. They are designed to taste, and as the case may be, melt just like the original food. You can even make a liquid butter substitute of your own with olive oil and a few drops of butter flavoring. Various seasonings may also be included as optional ingredients.

If the dairy products in ice cream bother you, try this substitute. Peel, slice, and run ripe bananas through a blender and freeze in pint containers. Allow to thaw and enjoy. You can vary this treat by including chopped nuts, if you are not sensitive to them, or a few strawberries or strawberry flavoring. This makes an excellent substitute for a sundae.

Don't feel as though you will be robbed of protein or other essential nutrients if you abandon milk or other dairy products. You will receive them in adequate quantities in other fresh whole foods. For instance, some beans contain the same percentage of calories from protein as 2% milk. Broccoli and asparagus contain even more.

Where youngsters are concerned regarding milk, a good substitute for any child over 2 years old who can tolerate it is soy milk. If this fails, rice milk is another option, but because it contains considerably less protein, it is important to include other foods in the diet that are rich in protein.

In regard to infants, breast feeding is the best bet, provided the mother avoids any substances to which she may be allergic. This strategy may also play a role in preventing allergies later on. However, a health care provider should consulted when youngsters of this age are involved.

Wheat Fill-Ins

If you have an allergy to wheat, you will have to give up most breads. Fortunately, there are some varieties that are made from other grains that taste just as good. There are also a number of good alternatives for inclusion in recipes. They include millet, arrowroot, buckwheat and tapioca. These grains are also gluten-free, as is rice and corn.

Bear in mind that some grains *do* contain gluten and should be avoided by gluten-sensitive individuals. They are: barley, einkorn, emmer, farro, kamut, oats, rye, spelt, triticale and of course wheat. It should be stated, however, that the gluten in oats is of a different molecular structure and therefore in its pure state might not evoke the same reaction as the gluten found in other grains. In fact, you might not react to it at all.

Peanut Pinch-Hitters

Should you have an allergy to peanuts, all is far from lost. You may be able to tolerate other nuts, that are just as nutritious. It might not be as difficult to eliminate peanuts from your diet, however, as peanut butter. If you love peanut butter but don't suffer from an allergy to other nuts, try almond butter, cashew butter, macadamia butter or other similar products. They are just as good for spreading on bread, crackers, and the like. In fact, they offer an intriguing change from the usual. If you prefer, you can quite easily make your own nut butters. Any raw or roasted nut or seed, can be ground up in a food processor and be mixed with olive oil.

The Tree Nut Juggle

If tree nuts are your problem, you will be able to swap one for another in your diet, unless you react to all of them. The same goes for nut butters. In the event all tree nuts affect you, try substituting seeds such as sunflower or pumpkin seeds, either as themselves or as a seed butter. If all else fails, other worthwhile substitutes come in the form of beans. To make certain you are receiving a good source of unsaturated fat that nuts would ordinarily provide, include avocados and olives in your diet.

Soy Subs

If soy products get the blame for your allergy, there are some worthwhile soy-free, high-protein foods such as beans, peas and lentils that can be used as ingredients in main dishes. Grains, nuts and seeds are also excellent choices for providing protein.

The Option for Chocolate

As far as chocolate goes, all you can do is give it the boot if you are allergic to it and replace it with carob, a most fitting substitute. Carob flour can replace chocolate or cocoa in any recipe in an equal proportion, unless that recipe calls for melted chocolate, in which case 3 tablespoons of carob and 1 and one half tablespoons of oil should be exchanged for every ounce of the melted chocolate.

If you are temporarily eliminating chocolate from your diet to determine if it is a problem, use dark, unsweetened baker's chocolate when you reintroduce it into your diet. Milk chocolate or filled chocolates will throw off the test because you won't know whether you are reacting to the chocolate or to the dairy ingredients or fillings. For the same reason, don't use other chocolate confections such as candy bars that have nuts and a lot of other ingredients in them.

If chocolate is your problem, you'd also better stear away from its close relatives: cocoa, cola and karaya gum. Karaya gum, by the way, is often listed on labels as "vegetable gum."

Replacements for Caffienated Beverages

If coffee, tea or soft drinks are your problem, it may be because of caffeine. Substitute decaffeinated beverages. Even they will contain a trace of caffeine, but the amount is negligible. In the event you find you cannot drink decaffeinated brew, it could be because of the chemicals used to remove the caffeine. Try switching to herb tea or drink fresh fruit and vegetable juices.

The Alternative for Dried Fruits

If you should have a reaction to dried fruit, such as raisins or figs, it could very well be attributed to the sulfite that has been added. Sulfite agents commonly employed are sulfur dioxide, sodium bisulfite, sodium sulfite, potassium bisulfite, sodium metabisulfite, calcium sulfite, and potassium metabisulfite. These additives have even been known to release small concentrations of sulfur dioxide gas that can be inhaled while eating them, producing a potential respiratory irritant. Look for products labeled "unsulfured."

Supplanting Sugar

Any foods with refined sugar, whether labeled "sucrose," "fructose," "maltose," "dextrose" or otherwise should not be a part of the diet. Honey is a better alternative, but even it should be used sparingly and should never be fed to children under 1 year old to safeguard against infant botulism. The best bet for satisfying cravings for sweets is to consume plenty of fresh fruit. For purposes of cooking, if you substitute with honey, use one half cup of it for every cup of sugar ordinarily required, and deduct one fourth cup of liquid from any recipe in which the honey is substituted. For any recipe including the instructions "sweeten to taste," rather than using sugar or a liquid sweetener, try blending in a fresh or dried fruit of your choice.

Fish Fill-Ins

If you are allergic to fish or shellfish, there are a lot of protein-rich foods you can eat instead. Walnuts, hempseeds and flaxseeds are good choices, along with soyfoods. They all contain the omega-3 fatty acids available in fish. Avocados and olives will also help fill the protein bill. And, of course, there are always lean meats such as chicken and turkey.

Table 32

Substitutes For Common Allergy-Producing Foods

For Corn

When eating:	When cooking:
Oatmeal	Arrowroot
Flour tortillas	Brown rice syrup
Popped rice	Concentrated fruit juice
Rice	Maple syrup
Rice chips	Millet
	Molasses
	Potato starch
	Tapioca starch

For Eggs

When eating:	When cooking:
Avocados	Applesauce
	Baking powder
	Baking Soda
	Fruit juice
	Mashed bananas
	Water

For Milk

When drinking:	When cooking:
Soy milk	Soy milk
	Vegetable juice
	Water

For Wheat

When eating: When cooking:

Corn   Arrowroot
Oats   Buckwheat
Rice   Millet
                            Tapioca

For Peanuts

When eating: When cooking:

Beans   Tree Nuts
Tree nuts

For Tree nuts

When eating: When cooking:

Beans   Seeds
Seeds   (sunflower,
   (sunflower,   pumpkin, etc.)
   pumpkin, etc.)

For Soy

Beans
Lentils
Nuts
Peas
Seeds

Table 32—continued	
For Chocolate	
When eating:	When cooking:
Carob	Carob
For Fish and Shellfish	
Chicken	
Nuts	
Seeds	
Turkey	

Other Considerations Concerning Food

Be aware of these common cross-reactions involving food and specific kinds of pollen. Those sensitive to ragweed may also react to melons, bananas, sunflower seeds, honey and chamomile tea. (Chamomile is also found in certain cosmetics.) Persons with a mugwort pollen allergy often react to apples, celery, carrots, melons, chamomile tea and some spices. Those with a birch tree pollen allergy may have a problem with apples, cherries, carrots, peaches, plums, pears, peanuts, potatoes, spinach, walnuts, wheat, buckwheat and honey. Individuals suffering from an allergy to pine may react to pine nuts, and those reacting to hazel may not be able to eat hazelnuts, filberts, or cobnuts. Those sensitive to grass may be unable to ingest melons, oranges, Swiss chard, tomatoes or wheat. An allergy to pellitory pollen may induce a reaction in some who indulge in cherries or melon.

Cooking, however, will solve the problem by destroying the offending allergen.

Occasionally, a sensitivity can be so severe that a person doesn't even have to eat an offending food for it to affect him or her. Some with a birch pollen allergy, for instance, (somewhat akin to the way one would normally react to peeling onions) may react adversely to peeling or even scrubbing potatoes. Even breathing the fragrances of certain foods being cooked can affect one.

A few have gone so far as to touch a small amount of a suspected food to their face to see how their skin feels about it. If it causes a skin rash, it's a sure warning not to eat it.

Going on a Pesticide-Free Diet

If you have uncovered an allergy to pesticides, you will obviously need to avoid them as much as possible. You can't rely on washing and peeling to remove pesticide residues. Once a food is sprayed, it absorbs a certain amount of the chemicals used. The only way to eliminate these contaminants from your diet is to consume foods that have not been sprayed with any chemicals intended to kill insects or other pests.

Fortunately, more items are appearing on grocery store shelves that have been organically grown. Purchase as many of these products as you can. Give them first priority. Not only will it be healthier for you, it will contribute to sales and encourage producers of organically grown foods to keep their goods coming. If your local market doesn't have what you want, ask for it. That will likewise encourage the grocer to purchase these items.

There are several kinds of certified organic produce. Look for items marked simply "100% organic." This term is used for foods that have been grown without any pesticides or synthetic fertilizers. If the label states: "Made with organic ingredients," this does not mean that all of the ingredients used are organic. There are other choices, marked with the labels "integrated pest management" (IPM), "sustainable agriculture" and "transitional agriculture," but with them comes no guarantee that the foods are pesticide-free.

In the case of IPM and sustainable agriculture, the use of pesticides is combined with biologic methods. Levels may be lower, but not nonexistent. Foods marked "transitional" are those grown without pesticides, but on land where pesticides have been previously utilized in the past few years. There may still be some traces of pesticides in the soil.

Of course, there is one other way you can assure yourself of getting pesticide-free food. Grow it yourself by starting a home vegetable garden. If the right crops are matched with the right region and they are grown following the correct procedures, the rewards can be great. If you've never indulged in a homegrown tomato, you're in for a treat.

You can even enjoy a year-round supply of veggies if you freeze, can or dry your harvest. You might also consider the addition of fruit-bearing trees, such as fig trees or pear trees for your backyard. If you are not allergic to nuts, a pecan tree would be a good choice.

Chapter 15
What to Do About Water

It should be a simple task to determine if you have developed an allergy to something in your water. You may wish to begin by trying a few tricks. Run your tap for at least 30 seconds before putting the water to use. There might be some build up of lead or other substances where the water has been standing in the pipes and that will give it a chance to escape. Another way of allowing potentially harmful substances to free themselves is to store tap water in an uncovered glass container in the refrigerator overnight. Yet another idea is to boil the water for at least 30 minutes.

Bottled Water as a Substitute

If it becomes necessary, substitute bottled water for what you have been drawing from the tap. Try it for 4 or 5 days and see if your symptoms abate. If at all possible, purchase bottled water in glass containers. Plastic containers outgas a certain amount of chemicals into the water. If this does not seem to work, try switching brands, as some water sold on grocery shelves is stored in plastic vats prior to bottling. If worse comes to worse, make distilled water your selection. Most of the chemicals and particles in the distilling process are left behind. Keep in mind, however, that extended use of distilled water for drinking may create a problem of its own because you may be robbed too long of needed minerals found in other drinking water.

As a precaution against mineral deficiency, in this case, it might help to take in a pinch of sea salt every day.

Drinking Plenty of Water

We've so often been told if we are suffering from a cold to drink plenty of liquids. It's not bad advice, but those afflicted with allergies should concentrate on drinking as much water as they can, rather than just other fluids such as fruit juices and sports drinks. While these other beverages can be of benefit by thinning mucus, which can in turn help relieve congestion, none possess an equal hydrating effect to that of plain water.

Whatever kind you choose, don't just consider it for drinking purposes. You will have to use it for cooking and in extreme cases for washing your hands. Bathing in it, of course, is too far afield, so if you are chlorine-sensitive, several crystals of sodium thiosulphate added to bath water will change chlorine to chloride.

Water Filtration

To avoid the expense of bottle water, however, you might want to consider filtering your tap water. The ordinary charcoal filters won't be adequate though unless piggybacked with some other purification material, such as that of activated carbon. In fact, carbon alone is efficient at removing chlorine, as well as industrial contaminants and some pesticides. Foul tastes and odors are also expelled. The only disadvantage is that activated carbon filters must be replaced approximately every 3 weeks or after every 20 gallons of water has been drawn to prevent recontamination.

The small carbon filters that hook up to the faucet are more economical, but they don't perform as well the more expensive kind, which must be installed below the sink and attached to a separate faucet that bypasses the existing water line.

You can also use a water distiller, but it has two drawbacks. It is difficult to keep clean and it requires a large amount of water.

Chapter 16
Dealing with Household Chemicals

The next time you pour a strong-smelling cleanser in the toilet bowl or spray on a heavily scented dose of deodorant, ask yourself if you really need it. No kidding. We use far too many chemicals that are potential allergens, and there are plenty of environmentally friendlier substitutes available that are both inexpensive and effective for cleaning and personal care, as well as those applied for home improvement.

Allergy-Free Cleaning

How can you effectively clean your surroundings without potent allergy-producing formulas? Actually, the answer is simple. A few basic readily available products are all you need. Two of the most notable ones are baking soda and white distilled vinegar. Other useful cleaners are denatured alcohol, borax, cream of tartar, hydrogen peroxide, lemon juice, olive oil and washing soda. These can be used alone or in certain combinations.

• Baking soda (sodium bicarbonate), also known as bicarbonate of soda, is a great all-purpose cleaner. Mixed with water, it can be used on kitchen counter tops, sinks, bathtubs, toilets, floors and appliances.

- By the same token, vinegar is useful for the same applications because of its strong acidic nature. It should be diluted with at least an equal amount of water, however, and don't leave it (or any acidic substance) standing for lengthy periods in sinks or tubs because it can destroy their surfaces. It can be combined with baking soda, borax, or washing soda.

- Alcohol is useful for removing stains and cleaning glass. The denatured (or isopropyl) variety is better than rubbing alcohol because it does not contain excess water or perfumes. Remember though, that it is flammable.

- Borax is a natural, all-purpose powdered cleaner composed of boron, sodium, oxygen and water. It is recommended for everything from clothes washing to cleaning the bathroom tile. It serves as a bleach, detergent, deodorizer, disinfectant, mildew retardant and water softener. It is, however, toxic if taken orally.

- Cream of tartar is a white crystalline mineral used in medicine and for cooking. It functions as a cleaner for metals, toilets, and the like.

- Lemon juice can be substituted for vinegar. Its high acidic content eats deep into dirt and stains.

- Olive oil is excellent for polishing wood surfaces.

- Salt is an effective non-scratching abrasive.

- Washing soda (sodium carbonate) known to some as washing crystals or sal soda is a mineral that is effective for removing oil and grease. It's also an excellent water softener. It possesses caustic qualities, so those with sensitive skin may need to wear gloves when using it. Be warned, however, that it can scratch fiberglass.

Here are some ideas for specific chores.

Scouring the Oven

When you're stuck with cleaning the oven, a solution of baking soda and water will be helpful. Warm water is more effective. For tougher stains, substitute borax for baking soda. It will furnish more abrasiveness. If this is not enough, use washing soda, which is good for even more formidable stains.

It's better to make a habit of wiping out your oven each time you finished cooking. Use a moist cloth before the surface has completely cooled. Better yet, prevent spills in the first place by using adequate-sized containers, as well as a cookie sheet or piece of tin foil beneath the cooking food in the event there is an overflow.

Unplugging Drains

Have a clogged drain? Reach for vinegar. A cupful poured down the drain will likely be all you will need. Allow it to stand a while and it will eat away at the blockage.

To prevent clogs, keep grease and larger particles out of the drain, and as an extra precaution, pour boiling water down the drain at least twice a week.

Toilet Bowl Cleaning

Sinks and bathtubs are bad enough, but toilets are a big chore. All you need here is a cup of borax. Pour it in the bowl, scrub with a brush, and flush. You can also include one fourth cup of vinegar for an even more effective job.

Making Your Wash Come Out

When washing clothes, add borax to the machine as you would any detergent. Include table salt in the load for tougher jobs and to prevent colors from running. Adding one fourth cup of lemon juice or vinegar to the wash cycle will serve as a bleaching agent. Caution: borax is not recommended for wool.

Washing Dishes

If you are trapped into washing dishes by hand, a vegetable oil-based soap is a good choice. Another idea is to add salt, washing soda, baking soda or borax to hot dishwater. Allow non-aluminum pots and pans with stubborn buildup to soak. It is not recommended that you use washing soda, baking soda or borax on aluminum, as these substances will subject them to discoloation and eventual deterioration.

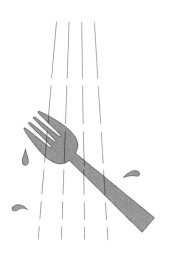

To clean coffee makers (non-aluminum only), fill to the top with water and add 1 teaspoon of borax per cup. Allow the coffee maker to go through the entire brewing cycle, then wait 20 minutes and rinse well. Tea kettles can be handled the same basic way. Just add the ingredients and boil for at least 10 minutes. For aluminum, use 2 tablespoons of vinegar per cup of water instead of borax.

Vegetable oil-based soaps, salt, washing soda, baking soda or borax can be used when washing dishes by hand.

If you are plagued by cups with coffee or tea stains, rub with a salt and vinegar paste. While you're at it, you may as well mix up the paste in one of the stained cups.

For cleaning nonstick cookware such as teflon, place 3 tablespoons of baking soda and 3 lemon slices in the soiled pot or pan and add enough water to cover the stains. Simmer on a flame until the stains have lifted. Then rinse thoroughly.

As a substitute for automatic dishwasher detergent, use borax. One-fourth of a cup will suffice. When cleaning the dishwasher itself, place 1 cup of vinegar into an empty dishwasher and run it through the cycle.

Polishing Your Furniture

You can concoct a polish by combining olive oil with lemon juice, and use it on the surfaces of coffee tables and other furniture. Just mix 2 parts olive oil with 1 part lemon juice in a glass jar and use whenever needed. It works on all wood surfaces.

Dealing with Spills

For cleaning spills on carpets, baking soda or borax comes into play. Sprinkle liberally on the affected area and rub in with a cloth. Allow it to sit overnight and vacuum the next day.

Brightening Up Glass

Mirrors, windows, and other glass objects can be cleaned with simple alcohol. Combine one fourth cup of alcohol for every quart of water in a bucket or spray bottle. Apply the contents with a sponge, then dry with a squeegee.

Shining Up Metal Items

Vinegar or lemon juice can be applied to chrome. Bronze, brass and copper can be cleaned with a mixture of lemon juice and salt. Hot ketchup is also effective.

Iron can be cleaned with olive oil.

Lemon and salt can be used for stainless steel, as can baking soda.

Tin can be cleaned using baking soda, borax, washing soda or cream of tartar.

Brighten up sterling silver with baking soda. A combination of baking soda, white toothpaste and warm water can be used for gold. Cream of tartar combined with vinegar works for aluminum.

Table 33

Substitutes for Commercial Cleaning Products

Oven cleaning	Baking soda, borax or washing soda
Drain cleaner	Vinegar
Toilet bowl cleaner	Borax or vinegar
Clothes detergents	Borax, lemon juice or vinegar
Dish washing soaps	Baking soda, borax, lemon juice, salt, vegetable oil-based soap or washing soda
Furniture polish	Olive oil and lemon juice
General spills	Baking soda or borax
Glass cleaner	Alcohol
Metal cleaners:	
Chrome	Vinegar or lemon juice
Bronze, brass, and copper	Lemon juice and salt, or hot ketchup
Iron	Olive oil
Stainless steel	Lemon and salt, or baking soda
Tin	Cream of tartar, baking soda, borax or washing soda
Sterling silver	Baking soda
Gold	Baking soda, white toothpaste and warm water
Aluminum	Cream of tartar and vinegar

A word of warning. Be cautious about using these cleaners on delicate fabrics. It you are uncertain about any material, test it first on a inconspicuous area. Some clothing, carpets or curtains can be damaged or discolored.

Even the use of these substances may not prevent an allergy, but they are much less likely to do so than those containing a lot of synthetic chemicals. If your skin is particularly sensitive, wear gloves while working.

Allergy-Free Personal Care

An allergy to a personal care item is far from the end of the world. Some products you can do without if need be, and there are several simple substitutes for some applications. Switching brands may also reduce, if not solve, the problem.

What to Do about Lipstick

If lipstick is your enemy, look for an unscented variety. Just eliminating the perfume found in other products of this nature could be enough to rescue you. If you prefer that "wet look" but are allergic to the lanolin in lip gloss, you might be able to get around the problem by applying petroleum jelly over the lipstick—if you don't adversely react to that.

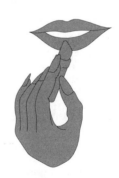

Using unscented lipsitck is a better choice for those who are allergic to cosmetics.

Giving the Cold Shoulder to Underarm Products

Commercial antiperspirants and deodorants don't have to be used at all. Don't laugh. This doesn't mean you have to leave a trail of body odor where ever you go. An application of baking soda under the arms works as well as anything else. Baking soda absorbs odors as well as a certain amount of moisture.

How to Handle Nail Polish

If you must use nail polish, apply it carefully in a well-ventilated area and avoid breathing the fragrance. Try not to make contact with the skin or cuticles. Wait until the polish has thoroughly dried before touching any part of your body.

Perfume Alternatives

You can concoct a homemade perfume by packing lavender or rose pedals in a jar of cold water and adding a tablespoon of lemon juice. Allow it to sit up for a couple of weeks, then strain it and apply.

About the only move you can make other than this if you want to wear commercial perfume or cologne is to experiment with different brands. The more expensive varieties are best beccause they are more likely to contain flower oils rather than man-made chemical materials.

Always apply any perfume sparingly and shower it off before retiring for the night.

Caring For Your Hair

For washing hair, here's an easy-to-make shampoo. Beat an egg in one pint of cool water and work it well into your hair. Then rinse in lukewarm water. Even if you react to eggs when eating them, you might not experience a problem when using them in this way. Baking soda can also be put to use as a shampoo. Apply a handful onto wet hair and rub into the scalp, then rinse. You won't produce any lather, but that doesn't mean your hair won't be clean.

For dandruff control, apply a half apple cider vinegar, half water solution to the scalp a few times a week before shampooing.

For a non-chemical hair spray, mix a one-eighth cup of powdered gelatin in one-eighth cup of cold water and heat in the top of a double boiler while stirring. Place the contents in a spray container. Store the unused portion in the refrigerator and heat before each use.

Semipermanent organic dyes and progressive dyes are least likely to illicit unpleasant reactions when it comes to hair dyes. Hair rinses are also a better choice. Hair dyes most likely to cause an allergic reaction are the oxidation kind. Of equal concern in this matter are the dyes containing the chemical paraphenylenediamine.

Mascara Considerations

To serve as mascara, try charcoal from a wood fire. If you use commercial brands of mascara, make an effort to minimize eye irritation, or to make it less likely in the first place, by applying it just shy of the corners of the eyes and only on the outermost portion of the lashes. Never apply liner to the inner part of the eyelid.

Giving Toothpaste and Mouthwash the Boot

There is a perfectly adequate substitute for both toothpaste and mouthwash. It's none other than baking soda. Apply it to your toothbrush as you would toothpaste or mix some in a glass of water and use as a gargle. A few drops of oil of peppermint can be added for flavor if desired. Avoid the use of salt, however, when brushing teeth. It's too abrasive for this purpose. Another way to freshen breath is to chew of a sprig of fresh parsley.

A Simple Alternative for After-Shave Lotion

Instead of after-shave lotion, just douse the face with cold water.

Face Cream Substitute

Mayonnaise can be used for a face cream. It is recommended by some beauty consultants and is good for dry skin. Even if you have experienced allergic reactions from the consumption of eggs, you might not react to this treatment.

A Better Eye Makeup Remover

Rather than relying on commercial eye makeup removers, use plain mineral oil. That way you will remove any exposure to fragrances that are included in the commercial product.

Treating Oily Skin

While mayonnaise works for dry skin, oily skin can be treated with orange juice. The juice from cucumbers or tomatoes also works.

A Natural Bath Powder

Try tapioca or arrowroot for a bath powder.

Table 34

Substitutes for Cosmetics	
After-shave lotion	Cold water
Antiperspirants/deodorants	Baking soda
Bath powder	Tapioca or arrowroot
Face cream	Mayonnaise
Hair care	Apple cider vinegar, baking soda, egg or powdered gelatin
Makeup remover	Mineral oil
Mascara	Charcoal from wood fire
Oily skin treatment	Cucumber juice, orange juice or tomato juice
Perfume	Lavender, or rose pedals and lemon juice
Toothpaste/mouthwash	Baking soda or oil of peppermint

As for soaps, purchase only those white in color and ones that are unscented and contain no antiseptics. Baby soaps are the safest as are those intended for washable woolens and fine fabrics.

Allergy-Free Home Improvement

Products used for home improvement are normally used less often, but that doesn't mean they can't and won't trigger an allergy. Fortunately, there are a number of choices when embarking on a project of this kind.

Alkyd-based paints seem to be better tolerated by most individuals than the latex variety. Latex may not seem as offensive odor-wise, but it often contains formaldehyde, synthetic rubber, acrylics, and preservatives such as biocide. Alkyd paints usually don't contain these things. However, they do include petroleum solvents, which can be a problem for some, at least until thoroughly dried. Epoxy paints are not recommended, because they can contaminate more heavily for longer periods of time. Casein paints, although they don't hold up as well, appear to be the best tolerated. However, they are formulated from milk protein and could prove trouble for those sensitive to milk. Even then, there are those who may not respond in the same way to a milk-based product that comes in contact with the skin or is inhaled as when ingesting milk or a food containing milk. Using lighter colors may help the cause. They contain less dye.

Whenever embarking on a painting project, plan it well. Do it at the time of year that fans can be put to use and windows can be opened. Don't use the central air system during this time, as this will only distribute the vapors to every part of the living quarters, as well as contaminate the ducts, fan, filter and other parts of the device. Brush paint on, don't rely on spraying. It is also a good idea to wear a respirator mask while work is in progress. (The kinds available from safety supply companies are generally better than those purchased at hardware stores.) A dust filter mask will be of no help where inhalation of fresh paint is concerned, because the vapors will come right through it as it is designed only to screen particulate matter. Wearing gloves is highly advised. Another idea is to plan a vacation for immediately after the task is completed. This will give the paint an opportunity to thoroughly dry, thereby completing most of its outgassing.

Any project involving paint, paint remover, varnish, or the like that can be moved out-of-doors, should be. For instance, if you plan to refinish a set of chest-of-drawers, at least transport them to the garage, and make sure the area is well-ventilated.

When using chemical sealers, make sure there is adequate ventilation. This especially holds true with silicone seal. It releases particularly strong vapors as it cures. Another product to be wary of is pipe joint compound, used for sealing threaded joints on natural gas lines.

Fortunately, as far as wood stains are concerned, for those willing to give it a try there is a satisfactory substitute. The ground shells of pecans or walnuts boiled in water will perform the same function without adding harmful vapors to the air.

As for glue, you might or might not have a choice about what kind to use, depending on the particular application, but where an option is involved, use a glue that emits the least amount of odor. That's a signal its outgassing is not as strong and not as many vapors are filling the air.

Take special care with any other chemicals that are necessary to use. Be as well-protected as you can and take the time to read and clearly understand the warning labels—and follow their instructions to the letter. Keep in mind, too, that even with commercial products that are labeled "non-toxic," there is no guarantee that no one will be affected by it.

And one final word. It is best to avoid aerosols. Instead of dispensing chemicals in this way, try adding liquid ingredients to pump-spray bottles when possible. The vapor will not be as fine and consequently less will remain airborne to be inhaled—and there won't be any propellants to worry about.

Chapter 17
Battling Pests the Safe Way

One must obviously be cautious when handling pesticides. They should never be used inside living quarters, and it is advisable to wear at the least a charcoal filter mask and gloves when applying lawn and garden pesticides. Make sure to dispense these products on a windless day or one in which only a mild breeze is blowing to minimize the chances of some of it from landing on your clothes or your neighbor's property.

All pesticides must be sealed properly after use and stored a secure place outside the house in their rightful container. A detached garage or storage shed is best. Apartment dwellers might consider a weatherproof box, which can be placed on a balcony or back porch.

But why bother with commercial pesticides at all? Most of your concern should be focused on the inside anyway, not the natural domain of these tiny crawling and flying creatures. There are safe, effective substitutes for handling many of the pests that so often plague us indoors.

Dealing With Ants

For exterminating most ants, honey and boric acid or borax thinly applied to small strips of paper can be effective. Initially this will attract them as they go after the sweet-tasting substance, but they will carry some of it back to the queen and eventually they will disappear.

The time it requires will be dependent upon the amount of nonpoisonous food supply they have already collected. (Warning: Although safer for the environment than synthetic pesticides, boric acid is still a poison and is harmful or fatal if swallowed, both for human beings and animals.)

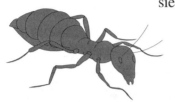

Another idea is to plant peppermint or pansies around doors and windows outside. They serve as good repellents. For fire ant mounds around the premises, carefully pour boiling water into them while wearing protective clothing. Remain as far away from the mound as possible and make a hasty retreat as soon as you have finished.

Boric acid and honey are effective for exterminating most ants.

Discouraging Beetles and Weevils

To prevent beetles or weevils from invading foodstuffs, store all vulnerable items, such as grains and flowers, in a cool spot in tightly sealed glass containers. Place a bay leaf in each container.

Chasing Off Fleas

Brewer's yeast can be added to your dog or cat's food to discourage fleas. They abhor the odor it gives off after the animal ingests it. Additionally, hot water and a mild, non-phosphate, biodegradable soap should be used to wash animal bedding frequently.

Pine needles placed in and around doghouses also work for fleas. Another effective measure is to salt the crevices of the doghouse. And remember not to neglect your pet's nutritional requirements. If a dog or cat should fall ill, it will be more prone to attack by fleas.

Natural Moth Busters

As far as moths are concerned, wash or brush infrequently worn clothes regularly. The insect and its eggs are fragile and cannot tolerate activity. For apparel that is to be stored for lengthy periods, wrap in paper and freeze a week or so prior to storing, then store in tightly fitting bags. If a mothball substitute is desired, try cedar wood shavings, blocks or balls.

Giving Roaches and Silverfish the Treatment

Boric acid is effective for roaches and silverfish. For roaches, sprinkle in corners, along baseboards, or where ever they are noticed. When dealing with silverfish, since they possess such a remarkable affinity for paper, mix the boric acid with flour and sugar and place it on strips of paper.

In addition, plain baking soda is toxic to roaches. Just mix a portion with an equal amount of sugar and distribute it. A simple formula for spraying can be made with 2 ounces of peppermint oil per gallon of water, or the same measure of eucalyptus oil can be used instead. Rosemary oil is another option, used in a ratio of 3 ounces per gallon of water.

In addition, roach traps that contain natural food bait and no insecticide can be used not only for roaches, but for a number of other crawling insects.

Getting Cockroaches Drunk

Strangely, roaches hold a remarkable affinity for beer. So why not open a bar for them? Try soaking a rag in some stale brew and put it on the kitchen floor overnight. They will likely get intoxicated enough to lose consciousness. Then they can be easily disposed of the next day.

Dealing With Flies

Basil plants grown around doors and windows will help repel flies. If necessary, hang flypaper (which can be made by applying a thin coat of honey to yellow paper) or use outdoor "zappers." Flies can also be repelled by hanging clusters of cloves in the affected area.

Repelling Mosquitos

The breeding of mosquitos should be prevented by emptying any stagnant water on the premises. If they are still a problem, grow basil plants around doors and windows or use outdoor "zappers."

Keeping the Upper Hand on Lice

If lice become a bother for dogs or cats, the adult insects can be controlled by the simple use of soap and water.

Parting with Ticks

Ticks are immune to many insecticides, making them somewhat more of a challenge. They can be removed from their host by swabbing them with rubbing alcohol and then pulling them off with tweezers when their heads come out of the skin. Be sure and wait until the process is complete, however, because if these insects get crushed before they have surfaced, some of the mouth parts may remain embedded in the skin.

Tackling Termites

For termites, another particularly formidable insect, there is no adequate substitute. It is advised that one limit the quantity of pesticide used by just spraying the nest directly. Cryolite is the best chemical to use. Although it is highly toxic, it produces a small amount of fumes.

If building a new home, institute preventative measures by making sure your contractor employs termite shields; *i. e.*, protects all wood near your foundation with sheet metal. Also, pressure-treated lumber can be used to prevent termite infestation.

Showing Mice Who's Boss

Mice can be dealt with by putting mousetraps to work. It is customary to bait them with cheese, but you can get more creative. Bacon or chocolate can usually also be used. If one bait fails, try another. To prevent their entry, try to locate the entrance sites and block those with an enduring substance such as steel wool or metal.

Also, a poison can be concocted that poses less hazard to children and pets. Make a mixture of one part flour, one part plaster of paris, and a dash of cocoa powder and sugar and sprinkle in areas where mice are sure to find it. This also works for rats if preferred over rat traps.

Of course, one should not lose sight of the fact that many pest problems in the home can be reduced or eliminated by maintaining clean habits. Ants are attracted by sugar and grease. Roaches adore all kinds of food remnants, as do flies. And, needless to say, everyone knows what can be the consequences of leaving wood piles lying around outside near the house, or inviting a tick-infested pet in.

Table 35

Pesticide Substitutes

Ants	Honey and boric acid or borax, peppermint plants or pansies
Beetles and weevils	Bay leafs
Fleas	Brewer's yeast, pine needles, salt
Flies	Basil plants, cloves, flypaper (honey applied to yellow paper) or outdoor "zappers"
Lice	Soap and water
Mice	Mousetraps baited with cheese, bacon, or chocolate; or poison composed of flour, plaster of paris, cocoa powder and sugar
Mosquitos	Basil plants or outdoor "zappers"
Moths	Cedar wood shavings, blocks or balls
Roaches and silverfish	Baking soda or boric acid or peppermint oil, eucalyptus oil or rosemary oil
Ticks	Alcohol

Chapter 18
Living with Pets

It's a sad affair, indeed, if you have to give up a pet because you or one of the family has developed a serious allergy to it. But before you surrender to this last resort, there are a number of moves that might ease or solve the problem.

Handling Dogs and Cats

If you are dealing with a dog or cat, keep it off the carpet. Carpets attract and harbor far too much debris and can easily become overloaded with dander and hair. By rights, dogs and cats should be banished to the yard. Not only will this move improve the condition of the indoor environment, but it will also curb the animal's shedding. This is because light has a bearing on the shedding process. In outside conditions, a dog or cat will only shed 2 times a year—in fall and late spring. If they are allowed to remain in the house, where electric lights are invariably turned on as soon as it gets dark, the shedding will continue year-round.

Additionally, it is a good idea to wash hands after petting or better yet, avoid direct contact. Grooming should be done by someone in the family who is not sensitive. Your animal should be brushed 2 or 3 times a week. This practice works wonders for keeping them clean. Use a soft brush, though. Stiff ones will scrape the skin and release more dander.

Another idea is to wipe the pet down with a wet towel. This is a good way to remove much of the saliva and loose hairs. Even a moist hand rubbed over a short-haired animal will pull out a surprising number of hairs.

Also, the pet should be shampooed at least every week or so. This can remove as much as 85% of the dander. Dogs can often be enough of a problem when it comes to a bath, but cats are worse, unless they are very young. A good strategy is to give the animal a treat just before and just after washing it. Hopefully, that will condition it well enough to make your experience tolerable. Use a veterinary shampoo, as the animal's skin is not designed for the harsher formulas produced for human scalps. This measure will, of course, place less strain on sensitive airways passages, as stronger shampoos will release more chemical vapors.

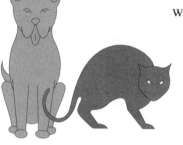

The coat can even be made nonstatic by rinsing it with a solution of 1 teaspoon of fabric softener in a quart of water. But watch out for chemical sensitivity. Fabric softeners contain perfumes and other ingredients that could be troublesome for some individuals.

Dogs and cats should be kept off carpeting and groomed regularly.

Don't forget to wash bedding frequently. This could be done after the animal is bathed each time. It will be easier to remember that way and the pet will start out fresh with a clean bed.

If you live in a conducive area, avoid kitty litter, which usually contains potent deodorants and train your cat to go outside. If you do use kitty litter, pour it into a metal pan rather than one made of plastic and change the litter frequently. Baking soda can be added to control odor. If odor is a particularly severe problem, consider changing your cat's diet.

Here is something else to consider. Most authorities agree that animal dander problems can be minimized by proper nutrition. (This also makes them less prone to attack by fleas). Going into detail about canine and feline diet is beyond the scope of this book, but pet owners should make sure their animals are getting properly balanced meals. Check with your veterinarian.

Don't neglect you own nutrition, either. You may be reducing your resistance and placing yourself wide open for a pet allergy you might not ordinarily have by maintaining poor eating habits.

And remember that it may not be the animal creating the allergy, but something associated with it, such as a flea collar, flea powder or kitty litter. It's worth investigating.

Table 36

Discouraging Dog and Cat Allergies

- Keep them off carpeting
- Wash hands after petting or avoid direct contact completely
- Brush regularly with soft brush
- Wipe down coat with wet towel
- Bath regularly using a veterinary shampoo
- Wash bedding frequently
- Housebreak animal
- Use metal pans for kitty litter
- Make sure they receive proper nutrition

Horse Sense

In regard to our equestrian friends, any nonallergic person who has been horseback riding should change his or her clothes before coming back indoors to protect one that is sensitive to this kind of animal. It's also a good idea for the person to take a shower as soon after the excursion as possible.

Plaster and Horsehair

The plaster in some old houses may contain horsehair. To find out if this is so, remove electrical switch covers and examine the plaster carefully. If you do detect horsehair, you might be able to reduce the level of allergens that escape into the air by repairing all cracks and holes.

How to Deal with Smaller Animals

As for our feathered friends and smaller animals such as hamsters, their saving grace may lie in the fact that they are usually confined to a single room, which limits to some degree the spread of any airborne allergen associated with it. About all one can do, however, if an allergy persists is to clean cages thoroughly and keep them clean. If appropriate, cages can be moved outside. Those affected, of course, should not make direct contact with the pet.

With regard to aquatic pets, keep fish tanks clean. The inside of tanks just above the water line attracts dust mites because of the fish food residues that accumulate there. Check for leaking filters too. This is an open invitation for mold. If you suspect an allergy to algae, keep the tank away from direct sunlight to discourage its proliferation and consider purchasing fish that eat algae. If you are allergic to mold, however, the fish tank should be placed in a position so it *does* get plenty of light, as mold loves dark places.

Chapter 19
Avoiding Bites and Stings

There are a number of ways to avoid insect bites and stings. Some you might never have considered; some are common sense. Here's the rundown.

Warnings about Bees and Wasps

As for bees and wasps, avoid nests by staying away from places where they are active, such as flower gardens. Also be especially observant when engaged in such activities as hedge trimming in case there is a hidden nest in your path. Do not wear loose clothing because the insects can more easily become entangled in them—and fly into a rage. For this same reason, long hair should be tied up.

Also avoid brightly colored attire. Khaki, tan, light green and white are the safest shades. Never crush a bee in proximity of its nest, as this could release an odor that signals the colony to swarm out in revenge. Don't douse yourself with perfume or cologne. Avoid flailing your arms or running away if a bee is approaching. Quick movements will likely startle the insect and inspire it to sting.

If a bee should land on you, try blowing at it gently. This will more likely encourage it to move along without startling it. If a bee gets caught in your clothing or hair, calmly crush it and high-tail it away from any nearby nest.

If you *are* stung, avoid slapping motions. Such a movement, combined with the scent discharged from a stinging bee might alert some of his friends, causing them to attack. Refrain from going out-of-doors barefoot and avoid open shoes. Don't drink soft drinks or eat sweet treats outside during warm weather. They attract bees and wasps. Note: Don't depend upon insect repellents. They are ineffective against stinging insects.

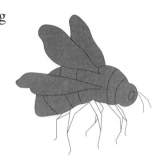

Those allergic to bee venom should avoid brightly colored attire, refrain from using perfume or cologne, and resist consuming sweet drinks and food out-of-doors.

Ducking Out on Spider Bites

To avoid spider bites, allow light to enter dark areas as much as possible. Use a broom to destroy spider webs. Don't give them a place to hide. Remove items such as piles of old clothing or newspapers in garages, attics or basements. Wear gloves when handling piles of rocks, lumber or the like. Shake out any bedding or clothing that has gone undisturbed for long periods before putting it to use. Inspect areas where spiders are likely to build a web, such as baseboard corners and closets and vacuum them when necessary.

Exercising Caution with Ants

Keep arms and legs covered. They are the most frequent targets for ants. Avoid all anthills. If you are sting by fire ants, avoid scratching to reduce the risk of blisters becoming infected.

Biting Back at Mosquitos

As far as mosquitos are concerned, as stated previously, discourage them by eliminating any standing water in the area. That's where mosquitos lay their eggs. Keep containers empty, as well as other items not usually intended to hold water, such as trash can lids. Also check for outdoor water leaks, repairing them if necessary, and make sure your drainage is adequate.

Don't sit outside at dusk when mosquitos are most active. Keep as much of your skin area covered as you can. The less surface area that is exposed, the less there is for a hopeful mosquito to attack. Avoid the use of perfume or cologne, which can attract them as it does other flying insects.

Keeping the Bedbugs from Biting

In regard to bedbugs, be vigilant. They can often be spotted in the seams of a mattress. Use your sniffer as well. An infested area tends to have a subtle odor that resembles that of cucumbers. Never leave dirty clothing on the bed or hanging nearby and be diligent about washing them. Reduce the number of places where they can hide by removing clutter from the bedroom. The same strategy goes for bedbugs as it does for mosquitos: Give them less area to attack by sleeping in long-sleeved and long-legged pajamas.

And here's something you may not think about. Bedbugs can enter a home by way of luggage. If you have just returned from a trip, vacuum your luggage before returning it to the inside. Also wash all your travel attire in hot water—and this includes anything you did not wear. It's best the discard your mattress if bedbugs are spotted, since eliminating an infestation from it is almost impossible. You should then wash all bedding at once in hot water.

Table 37

Averting Bites and Stings

Bees and Wasps

- Avoid nests
- Don't wear loose clothing
- Tie up long hair
- Avoid brightly colored attire
- Never crush a bee in proximity of its nest
- Avoid using perfume or cologne
- Avoid rapid motions
- If stung, avoid slapping motions
- Refrain from going out-of-doors barefoot and avoid open shoes
- Don't drink soft drinks or eat sweet treats outside

Spiders

- Allow light to enter dark areas as much as possible
- Use a broom to destroy spider webs
- Remove items where they can hide
- Wear gloves when working out-of-doors
- Shake out any bedding or clothing that has gone undisturbed for long periods
- Inspect areas where spiders are likely to build a web and vacuum them when necessary

Ants

- Keep arms and legs covered
- Avoid all anthills

Mosquitos
_____

• Eliminate standing water in the area
• Don't sit outside at dusk
• Keep as much of your skin area covered as you can
• Avoid using perfume or cologne

Bedbugs
_____

• Check mattresses
• Never leave dirty clothing on the bed or hanging nearby
• Remove clutter from the bedroom
• Sleeping in long-sleeved and long-legged pajamas
• If you have just returned from a trip, vacuum your luggage
  before returning it to the inside
• Wash all travel attire in hot water
• Discard your mattress if bedbugs are spotted and immedi-
  ately wash all bedding in hot water

Chapter 20
Taking your Medicine

It's so easy to do. You awaken with a stuffy nose and reach for a decongestant. You feel the pounding of a headache as an afternoon of work wears on and you go for an aspirin. You toss and turn for hours trying to nod off and finally give in to a sleeping pill. Sometimes, however, the "modern miracles" medical science has provided may sometimes be more of a curse than a godsend. If symptoms are relieved, well and good. But if a drug triggers an allergic reaction, especially a severe one, it's quite another story.

There will be no attempt here to offer specific advice on the matter of prescription drugs. That must be left to the physicians. It only bears saying that you should report any unexpected reactions from such medication to your doctor. He or she may be able to prescribe a different remedy that you can tolerate.

This first thing you should ask yourself before regularly relying on over-the-counter medication—for that matter prescription drugs as well—is: "What could be causing my symptoms?" If you are able to stop what's manufactering the problem, you won't require the medicine in the first place. For example, let's say your are stricken with a bad case of hay fever on certain afternoons. If you think the matter through, you might realize it could be attributable to the lawn mowing job you perform shortly prior to each attack. Or if you are beset by an upset stomach before bedtime some nights, you might be able to trace it to the unusually large helpings of ice cream you have been having for dessert at dinner. The solution might be as simple as wearing a dust mask when doing yard work or changing a few eating customs.

Advice About Using Medications

If you must take any over-the-counter remedies, examine labels carefully, become familiar with the ingredients, apprise yourself of the possible side effects, and as the ads always proclaim, "use only as directed."

Here are a few additional tips. Taking products in powder form is generally better than swallowing tablets. There are more inactive ingredients contained in tablets, such as coatings and binders. Even gelatin capsules can prove troublesome for some, as they may be made of potentially allergenic foods such as pork or beef. So if using a product in this form, the safest move is to empty the capsule and just take the contents.

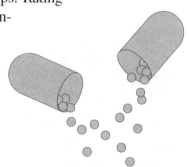

To guard against an allergic reaction to gelatin from medications in capsule form, pull apart the capsule and take the contents only.

To guard against the possibility of error, never takes medicine in the dark. Try to get by on the smallest dose you can. Never transfer medications from their original container. Keep medications tightly sealed and never remove the label. Store them away from direct heat and sunlight. Keep them out of reach from children. Don't allow liquid medications to freeze. Do not use a medicine cabinet to store drugs, as moisture or heat may cause them to break down. Any medications that are outdated or no longer required should be discarded, unless otherwise directed, by flushing them down the toilet.

Home Remedies for the Allergy Prone

If you're seeking temporary relief from troublesome common conditions and want to be safer from allergy, however, there are a number of simple home remedies that can be put into action.

Antacid

For an antacid to relieve acid indigestion, upset stomach or heatburn, try baking soda. Place one-half teaspoon in a 4 ounces of water, stir and drink. Take every 2 hours, if necessary, or as directed by your doctor. Do not exceed the recommended dosage stated on the label and consult your healthcare provider before use if you are on a sodium restricted diet or contact him or her if severe stomach pain occurs after taking this product.

Arthritis Pain

To retard the progression of arthritis and alleviate pain brought on by it, take 1 teaspoon of apple cider vinegar in a glass of water 4 times a day.

Asthma

Asthma, according to some medical practitioners, may alleviated by holding vinegar-soaked pads on the inside of wrists. Another solution which may help for milder attacks of asthma involves stirring a teaspoon of apple cider vinegar in a tumbler of water and taking the solution in sips for 30 minutes. Wait one half hour and repeat the procedure. This entire sequence can be repeated if necessary. The simple matter of drinking plenty of warm liquids will help thin mucus in the lungs so it can more easily be discharged by coughing. This also produces a relaxing effect on the bronchial muscles.

Constipation

Constipation can be relieved by prunes, figs or bran. Just a small amount of any will often be enough. Epsom salt is also effective.

Coughs

Whenever plagued with a tickling cough, sip on a cup of comfrey tea.

Diarrhea

Diarrhea can be alleviated with garlic. Take a teaspoonful of diced garlic with honey 2 or 3 times a day. Garlic is good for other intestinal ailments as well.

Fatigue

A suggested treatment for chronic fatigue comes from the renown Dr. Earl Mindell, author of a number of excellent health books. At bedtime, take 3 teaspoons of apple cider vinegar to an eighth cup of honey. Vinegar is capable of nullifying the effect of lactic acid in the bloodstream, which can cause fatigue when released in excess amounts due to exercise or stress. Meanwhile, the honey provides extra energy.

Food Poisoning

For alleviating symptoms produced by food poisoning, take a quarter teaspoon of apple cider vinegar once a day until the poison is neutralized.

Hay Fever

In regard to symptoms in general brought on by hay fever, comfrey has been reported to help control them. The most effective method to employ is that of ingesting fresh leafs from the plant. Since the leaves are hairy, make them more palatable by folding them up into small pieces. The next best alternative is to brew comfrey tea.

Headaches

Some headaches can be relieved by pouring a dash of apple cider vinegar into the water in an electric vaporizer and breathing the vapors for 5 minutes. If a vaporizer is not available, mix 2 teaspoons of apple cider vinegar with 2 cups of distilled water and pour into a pan. Heat it to a boil. Remove it from the stove as the steam begins to rise, then begin breathing the vapor. For maximum effect, drape a towel over the head to trap the steam. Breath carefully at first to avoid burning yourself.

Another solution for headaches: Squeeze some garlic juice into a teaspoon of honey and eat it. You may also find relief by drinking chamomile tea or peppermint tea. To keep headaches away, medical experts say to eat a lot of raw spinach. It is loaded with an enzyme that breaks down headache-causing chemicals.

Hiccups

To halt hiccups, slowly sip on a glass of warm water in which 1 teaspoon of apple cider vinegar has been added. Or drink tea made from dill leaves.

Leg Cramps

For leg cramps, relief may be achieved from a glass of water combined with 1 or 2 teaspoons of apple cider vinegar.

Morning Sickness

In regard to morning sickness, add a teaspoon of apple cider vinegar to a glass of water and drink it just after awakening.

Muscle Soreness

To relieve the discomfort of muscle soreness, try dipping a cloth in apple cider vinegar, wring it out, and apply it to the affected area. This works for sprains too. If the problem is not localized, pour 3 cups of apple cider vinegar into a bathtub filled with warm water, then soak in it.

Nasal Congestion

Nasal congestion brought on by sinusitis may be diminished by drinking a glass of water combined with a teaspoon of apple cider vinegar—to be repeated, if necessary, 6 additional times on an hourly basis.

Relief may also be achieved merely by inhaling steam. For more effectiveness, use a heated mixture of one part vinegar and one part water vapor. A small amount of eucalyptus oil can be added to the water instead of the vinegar or you can place several eucalyptus leaves (available at many health food stores) in a pot of water and boil for 5 minutes, then remove from the heat and breath the vapors. Discontinue use, however, if the nasal passages seem irritated. Just inhaling hot humid air helps unblock the sinus cavity, as well as reduces the reaction that transpires when an allergen gains entrance to the nose.

Diced garlic taken with water also helps the cause. Another idea is to take a bite of hot pepper, such as jalapeno or chile, if you can stand it, or incorporate it into your food. Horseradish can also be effective. Add 1 teaspoon of freshly grated horseradish and a teaspoon of honey to a glass of warm water and drink. The honey will force the horseradish to stick to the back of the throat, which stimulates your

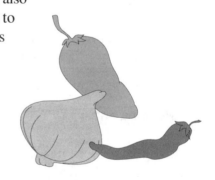

Eating pungent foods such as garlic and hot peppers can often diminish nasal congestion.

sinus passages and lungs to produce more mucus. The mucus, in turn, will help eliminate the allergen responsible when it is discharged by blowing your nose. This can also be used as a gargle if you don't desire to drink it. Don't use this remedy, however, if you suffer from chronic stomach inflammation or a kidney disorder.

Also, a saline solution (available at any pharmacy) can be poured into a dropper bottle and squirted in the nose as often as needed. If you don't prefer treatment administered in this way, a nonmedicated saline gel applied just inside the nose can help, and it holds the added advantage of trapping pollen and other particulate matter, preventing it from penetrating farther into the nose.

Runny Nose

For a runny nose, sage tea can come to the rescue because it has a drying effect. It may be taken as much as 6 times daily. Sage has additional advantages. It can help prevent infections that often result from chronic allergies. It is also capable of strengthening the immune system, which could help prevent allergies from worsening. To be effective, however, sage, as with all herbs, must be stored in an airtight glass container in a cool, dark place to preserve freshness. This warning, however: Do not use it if you are pregnant, nursing, hypoglycemic or undergoing anticonvulsant therapy.

Sore Throat

For a sore throat, whether caused by a virus or bacteria, add a tablespoon full of apple cider vinegar to a glass of warm water and use as a gargle. Repeat as needed. If a more potent formula is required, make the mixture 1 part vinegar and 1 part water. Do not swallow the liquid, however, because the vinegar draws out throat germs from the tissues. This formula can be applied for laryngitis as well.

Sucking on a clove of garlic also works. Just scrape it with your teeth occasionally to release some of the juice. You can chew it, but this tends to induce a burning sensation that some people may not like.

Insect Bites and Stings

For insect bites and stings, apply undiluted apple cider vinegar to the affected area as soon as possible to arrest pain and relieve itching. This practice is now endorsed by the Medical Journal of Australia as well as a number of other organizations. Apple cider vinegar will also neutralize the venom of jellyfish.

Also, honey dabbed on the area will ease pain and reduce swelling from stings, as will wheat germ oil. Meat tenderizer can also be applied. Aloe vera gel will help too. Soak a cloth with it and bind it on to the wounded area or better yet, split an aloe vera leaf and apply the pulp. Warning: Aloe vera interacts unfavorably with steroid tablets. Swelling can also be reduced by the application of a cold ice pack or ice wrapped in a cloth.

Note: In cases of any stings inflicted by an insect with a stinger, don't attempt to remove it by pulling. Doing so will squeeze more venom into the wound. Instead, scrape the stinger out of the skin with a dull knife or your fingernail.

Bleeding

Halt bleeding faster by pressing a cotton swab moistened with apple cider vinegar on cuts and abrasions. Although the acidic content of the vinegar will create a burning sensation, it aids in congealing the blood as well as reduces the chance of infection. For best results, swab the wound with more apple cider vinegar every day until the skin returns to normal.

Inflammation

It is possible to relieve inflammation with a "vitamin C bath." Just add 3 tablespoons of ascorbic acid powder to a warm bath and soak.

Some of the vitamin C will be absorbed into the skin. Ascorbic acid powder can be found in most health food stores.

Nosebleeds

To stop nosebleeds, gently stuff a cotton ball soaked in apple cider vinegar up one or both nostrils. Sit down and relax, then while breathing though the mouth, pinch the nose. Continue five to ten minutes. Then gently remove the cotton. Repeat if necessary.

Burns

Honey works for burns. Apply it liberally to the stricken area. Ironically, apple cider vinegar does not create a burning pain when applied to minor burns themselves. It actually subdues the pain. Simply administer it to the wound directly from the bottle by patting it on the affected portion of skin. In this case it doesn't even have to be diluted. Repeat every twenty minutes or so. Note: If the vinegar is cold, it tends to be more effective. Garlic oil is also good for burns. Just rub the oil from a punctured garlic oil capsule into the affected area for swift pain relief.

Apple cider vinegar works for sunburn as well. Gently sponge on the affected portion of the skin. If larger surface areas have been affected, add 1 or 2 cups of apple cider vinegar to a bathtub full of cool water and take a plunge. After bathing, apply another round of apple cider vinegar to appropriate areas.

Cold Sores

Remove the discomfort of cold sores and hasten their healing by applying undiluted apple cider vinegar to the affected area.

Dandruff

Don't let dandruff ruin your day. Sometimes bacteria will clog hair follicles which in turn produces this annoying condition. Fortunately, the enzymes as well as the acid contained in apple cider vinegar will kill the bacteria. Massage your scalp several times a week with undiluted apple cider vinegar just before shampooing. Not only can this help to eliminate dandruff, it's good for the hair.

Ear Problems

For earaches, puncture a garlic oil capsule, pour it into the ear, and stuff it with cotton. This can become effective in as little as 15 minutes.

An old folk remedy suggests that diluted apple cider vinegar placed in the ears will prevent an ear infection. Studies tell us that this may be valid. Simply mix the vinegar with an equal portion of distilled water or alcohol and use an ear dropper for application. This procedure is also helpful for swimmer's ear.

Some have reported relief from tinnitus by depositing onion juice in their ears. Apply it as needed.

Foot Problems

Here are some solutions for foot problems. For relief of pain from minor injuries, soak feet in a pan of hot water and Epsom salt.

The all-too-common athlete's foot can be relieved by soaking feet in a mixture of one part vinegar and one part lukewarm water. This should be done for at least 10 minutes once or twice each day until symptoms subside. Another solution is to rinse the feet several times a day in apple cider vinegar.

The pain and swelling of blisters have been reported to be relieved by massaging garlic oil into the feet.

Dissolve corns and callouses by soaking them in a pan of warm water and one third cup of vinegar for approximately one half hour.

Then rub the affected area with a coarse towel. Next rub more gently with a pumice stone. Finally, apply a gauze bandage soaked with nothing more than apple cider vinegar and leave overnight. Change the bandage and continue use the next day.

From Toe to Head

Your nasal allergy symptoms can be decreased by soaking your feet in warm water—or so medical evidence suggests, based on a study conducted at the University of Chicago involving people with seasonal allergic rhinitis. After being exposed to doses of their allergens, their feet were immersed either in warm water or water at room temperature for 5 minutes before as well as during each exposure. It was discovered that those soaking their feet in warm water experienced notably reduced symptoms compared to those who did not.

Hives

For hives, apply a paste made from apple cider vinegar and cornstarch to the affected skin. As this paste begins to dry it will draw out the toxins that are causing the itching.

Poison Ivy

In the case of poison ivy, a solution of 1 part apple cider vinegar and 1 part distilled water administered to the affected area will diminish itching and reduce swelling. This works out not only for poison ivy but for its relatives poison oak and poison sumac as well. Lemon juice is also effective. Simply slice a lemon and rub it into the stricken area.

Ringworm

Apple cider vinegar can be an effective treatment for ringworm—in actuality a fungus that is transmitted from child to child or from animal to child. With the fingers, apply it undiluted to the scalp at the infested area. Repeat at least five more times throughout the day until the problem clears up.

Toothaches

Rub oil of cloves on the surrounding gum area.

General Itching

To relieve itching in general, use ice packs or cool compresses. Even a simple ice cube rubbed on the affected area will help. For a widespread problem, a bath of lukewarm water and 2 cups of cornstarch can be effective. As a substitute for cornstarch, colloidal oatmeal can be used—or both can be combined. Caution: This will likely make your tub slippery, so be extra careful.

General Respiratory Difficulties

For respiratory difficulties in general, it is important to include plenty of vitamin C in your diet. It acts as a natural antihistamine. The best source of vitamin C is citrus fruit. Make it a habit to eat an orange or grapefruit everyday. That will normally give your body all the vitamin C it needs. If one doesn't seem to be enough, try doubling up. You might want to have a grapefruit for breakfast and include an orange with your noontime meal. Feel free to try even more. Other vitamins, minerals and enzymes are also important. A sound diet with plenty of fresh fruits, vegetables, legumes and grains might very well be what is needed to halt nagging symptoms, if not prevent them—allergic or otherwise.

Hay fever, for example, may be prevented by consuming plenty of apples, onions, leaf lettuce, kale, cranberries, citrus fruit and buckwheat. They contain a bioflavonoid called quercetin, which serves as a natural antihistamine. Yellow onions supply the richest source.

Warning: Some foods interact in different ways with certain drugs. Asthmatics using theophylline, for instance, should not indulge in meals containing cruciferous vegetables such as broccoli, Brussels sprouts, cabbage, cauliflower and kale, as well as charcoal-grilled meats, as they can cause your body to more quickly eliminate the medicine. If you have to be on certain prescription medications such as astemizole (Hismana) or fexofenadine (Allegra), you may not be able to eat grapefruit. This fruit will enhance the absorption of all that the body ingests—including any drugs taken. That might wallop you with the effects of a bigger dose. In addition, side effects from the medicine could increase. This is especially true with sage, which can boost the sedative side effects of certain drugs.

In addition, herbal medicines may cross-react with certain kinds of pollen if they contain related plant materials. It is advisable that, if at all possible, you find out the ingredients used for any of these remedies and see whether any of them belong to the same plant family as the pollen in which you are allergic.

One additional note: Stinging nettle has been reported to be a natural alternative to allergy prescription drugs. A study conducted by the National College of Naturopathic Medicine revealed that 58% of those taking stinging nettle said they achieved moderate or excellent results after only 1 week. It is available in capsule form at health food stores. However, it may actually cause symptoms to increase in rare cases, so it is advisable to take only a small dose at first to test your reaction. If your doctor has prescribed allergy medication for you, check with him or her for advice in this matter.

Table 38

Substitutes for Over-the-Counter Medications

Antacid	Baking soda
Arthritis pain	Apple cider vinegar
Asthma	Apple cider vinegar
Constipation	Prunes, figs, bran or Epsom salt
Coughs	Comfrey tea
Diarrhea	Garlic and honey
Fatigue	Apple cider vinegar and honey
Food poisoning	Apple cider vinegar
Hay fever	Comfrey
Headaches	Apple cider vinegar, garlic juice and honey or chamomile tea or peppermint tea
Hiccups	Apple cider vinegar or tea made from dill leaves
Laryngitis	Apple cider vinegar
Leg cramps	Apple cider vinegar
Morning sickness	Apple cider vinegar
Muscle soreness	Apple cider vinegar
Nasal congestion	Apple cider vinegar, steam, eucalyptus oil or leaves, or diced garlic, hot peppers, horseradish and honey, saline solution or non-medicated saline gel
Runny nose	Sage tea
Sore throat	Apple cider vinegar, garlic
Insect bites and stings	Apple cider vinegar, honey, wheat germ oil, meat tenderizer or aloe vera gel
Bleeding	Apple cider vinegar

Inflammation	Ascorbic acid powder
Nosebleeds	Apple cider vinegar
Burns	Honey, apple cider vinegar or garlic oil
Cold sores	Apple cider vinegar
Dandruff	Apple cider vinegar
Ear problems	Earaches: Garlic oil
	Tinnitus: Onion juice
Foot problems	Pain from minor injuries: Hot water and Epsom salts
	Athlete's foot: Apple cider vinegar and warm water
	Blisters: Garlic oil
	Corns and callouses: Warm water, vinegar and pumice stone
Hives	Apple cider vinegar and cornstarch
Poison ivy	Apple cider vinegar and distilled water or lemon juice
Ringworm	Apple cider vinegar and distilled water
Toothache	Oil of cloves

Chapter 21
Selecting the Proper Clothing and Bedding

For allergy-prone individuals, clothing woven from natural fibers beats those containing synthetics. The best all-round fabric is cotton, but take heed. This material can be adulterated with toxic materials and sometimes it is combined with synthetic materials such as polyester. Beware of apparel labeled as "permanent-press," "wrinkle-free" or "wash-and-wear." Cotton that has been sized can makes problems too for sensitive persons. It can be coated with glues, starch and even shellac.

Very few have problems with silk or linen.

Unprocessed wool is also usually safe. Most of the cases of itching is not caused by allergy, but purely because of mechanical irritation. This problem can be reduced or stopped by layering wool clothing over cotton undergarments. Beware of treated wool, which contains shrink-proof chemicals and dye that might prove allergenic, although dyes contained in natural fibers seem to be more tolerated than those used for synthetic fabrics. If you react to this and untreated wool is unavailable, thick cotton sweaters and corduroy pants are good substitutes.

Socks are not to be overlooked either. All-cotton socks are in order for the sensitive. White is the best choice. The dyes used for colors may affect some, although fabric allergies from dyes are less common. If a reaction to dye *is* a problem, it's the darker colors that are of more concern. And even though they are largely colorfast, that doesn't mean some measure of the dye cannot be lifted off by perspiration. Try to change socks once during the day, particularly when the weather is warm. This also goes for shoes, if possible, especially if you've been exercising in them.

Don't forget about gloves, handbags, hats, belts, hose, suspenders, bras, garter belts and girdles. Search for chemical-free materials.

As for bedding, it should be cotton too. It is best for mattresses to contain cotton stuffing. As this is often a challenge to find, conventional mattresses and bedsprings can be encased in zipped cotton covers. A cover of this kind will serve as a barrier against fumes from foam rubber or other synthetics. Aluminum foil (shiny side up) may also be effective if used as a mattress cover. Cotton pads can be placed atop the mattress, which in turn can be overlayed with cotton sheets.

Wool is a good choice for blankets if it can be tolerated. Otherwise, try substituting thermal cotton blankets.

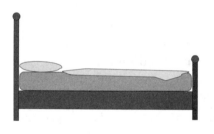

Bedding for allergic individuals should be composed of cotton, including mattresses if possible. Mattresses which are not cotton-stuffed can be encased in zipped cotton covers.

The best bet to serve as a pillow is rolled up cotton garments such as T-shirts stuffed into a cotton pillow case. Another good stuffer: cloth diapers.

In the worst case scenario, you might have to resort to an aluminum bed with springs in the form of a folding cot, layered with 100% cotton blankets to serve as a mattress. These blankets should be washed thoroughly in something basic such as baking soda.

And when shopping for natural fabrics, don't overlook curtains and rugs. They count too.

Fabric Tests

There are several ways fabrics can be tested to determine how safe they are for the allergy-stricken. That way you will have a better idea if what you have on hand is all right for you and be more able to identify what items are the best for purchase, especially if you are seeking the raw materials to make your own clothes.

One is the wrinkle test. Crush the material in question. If it wrinkles, it should be free of wrinkle-proof agents. As a general rule, the less an item wrinkles, the greater the amount of chemical treatment has been added.

The sniff test can also be of help. If you detect odors when closely smelling of a garment, you are probably getting a whiff of formaldehyde or other chemicals. The stronger the odor, the higher the concentration of chemicals probably are.

If your olfactory senses are not particularly acute, there are several variations to this test. Heat increases the outgassing process, so try ironing the material and sniffing it while still warm. You can also intensify an odor by wadding up small articles in a glass jar, tightening the cap, and leaving it closed for 24 to 48 hours before sniffing.

Bear in mind that apparel that has been stored near synthetic fibers may pick up odors from them, especially when new. Some clothes may have to be placed in different closets for sensitive individuals. If you are purchasing material intended for homemade attire in which you suspect this could be the case, obtain a small sample and take it home where you can test it after washing it and airing it out.

Also be aware that mothproofing is seldom declared on garment labels. This can often be detected if you notice an odor similar to dry-cleaning fluid that holds a hint of mothball odor.

The water test is another possibility, but it can only the used for cotton. Place a drop of water on the article. It will quickly be absorbed if the cotton is untreated. Otherwise, a small bubble will remain on the surface. The only exception to this: if the material is barrier cloth or a primitive fabric such as Mexican cotton or unbleached muslin. These possess a strong odor from the sizings, but they usually wash out easily.

The sense of touch may work for some. Place the palm of your hand lightly on a surface you know to be chemically uncontaminated and then put it on the article in question. Do not press heavily and do not rub. Rubbing will activate nerve endings that negate the skin's sensitivity to this test. You may be able to experience a tingly sensation or a crawley feeling. This could indicate a problem.

The Vinegar Treatment

If you find anything about a material that is bothersome, you may be able to solve the problem with apple cider vinegar. Pour two cups of it in a quarter tub of water. Make certain it is apple cider vinegar, not distilled. If washable woolens are involved, the water must be cold. For sheers, use warm water, and in the case of cottons the temperature should be hot. Soak, then wash thoroughly. Rinse and hang out to dry. Repeat the procedure if necessary.

Note: This will probably not be effective on mothproofed or permapress fabrics.

Hopefully, you are now armed with enough information to successfully deal with your allergy. Even if you must seek professional help, you will better be able to work with your doctor toward solving the problem. At any rate, good luck in bidding farewell to your allergy.

Appendix A

How to Handle an Allergic Emergency

Hopefully, neither you nor anyone you know will ever have to face a life-threatening reaction from an allergen. But if the occasion should arise, the following will help you to identify it for what it is and know what action to take for it. There are 3 potentially fatal conditions: anaphylaxis (the most common life-threatening reaction), and less typically but equally dangerous, laryngeal edema, and status asthmaticus (a severe form of asthma).

Initial symptoms characterizing anaphylaxis:

- Weakness
- Anxiety
- Dizziness
- Paleness
- Hoarseness
- Respiratory distress
- Collapse

These symptoms may be succeeded by any of the following:

• Runny nose (especially sudden)
• Wheezing
• Coughing
• Swollen vocal cords
• Bronchospasm
• Low blood pressure
• Rapid heartbeat
• Hives
• Swelling of the skin
• Skin discoloration (bluish tinge)
• Itching (especially of the face)
• Flushing (especially intense)
• Diarrhea
• Nausea
• Vomiting
• Stomach cramps
• Bloating

A reaction of this sort is attributed directly to histamine and other allergy-provoking substances released by cells that have been affected by the antibody-antigen reaction. Respiratory distress results from spasms in the muscular walls of the bronchi, which narrows the air passages. The drop in blood pressure (this in itself also known as anaphylactic shock) is the result of dilation of the small blood vessels.

Constricted airways are, of course, the greatest threat. The second greatest threat is low blood pressure.

The most common cause of anaphylaxis is penicillin. The second most common is insect stings. Also a threat are drugs (including aspirin), radiographic dye (employed as a medical diagnostic tool) and foods, such as fish and eggs.

Not all cases of anaphylaxis emerge immediately. Sometimes the symptoms will be delayed for an hour or two. However, there are most often initial signs preluding the condition, such as swelling or itching of the mouth, hoarseness, the sensation of a lump in the throat or stomach upset. This may be followed by more generalized symptoms, such as weakness, disorientation, feeling of warmth or overall itching.

Laryngeal edema is a swelling of the throat or windpipe. It can occur alone or accompany anaphylactic shock.

Status asthmaticus is characterized by:

• Weakness

• Fatigue

• Irregular heartbeat

• High pulse

• Bulging of the neck muscles

• Sweating

• Expanded chest cage

• Deepening of notch over breastbone

• Loud wheezing that stops

• Respiratory distress

• An attack unresponsive to routine treatment

• An attack that increases in intensity

• An attack that fails to improve

Needless to say, if any of the above conditions occur, immediate action is essential, just as with a heart attack. Put in a call for medical assistance at once if a telephone is available. In the meantime, it is important to reduce swelling and elevate blood pressure back to normal. Hopefully, an allergy kit or an adrenaline kit will be available. (Anyone with a history of severe allergy should have one.) These kits are equipped with adrenaline (epinephrine). Adrenaline should be administered as soon as possible. This is the most effective way to counteract severe attacks. Injecting adrenaline, however, requires medical instruction. If you don't know how, now's the time to learn. Your doctor can teach you how, or he or she can prescribe an adrenaline inhaler. Warning: Adrenaline cannot be used safely if you have a heart condition.

Allergy kits usually also contain antihistamine tablets. They can be of help to further neutralize the flood of histamine. However, you should know ahead of time how much you should take.

If applicable, you may have to administer a tourniquet. It is to be applied 2 to 4 inches above an insect sting toward the trunk of the body to retard the circulation that will, in turn, slow the circulation of venom. To be effective, it must be applied immediately. And a tourniquet is intended for the limbs only (arms and legs). Tie it firmly, but not so tightly that the circulation is completely cut off. It should be loosened about every 5 minutes. Keep in mind that it is designed for temporary use, until medical help becomes available.

If your medical kit does not contain a tourniquet, one can be fashioned out of a belt, cloth, rope or anything similar, including a dog leash.

If you haven't already done so, call for medical assistance or get the victim to a hospital, as additional treatment may be required. If you have been taking corticosteroids, inform the doctor because they could diminish your body's ability to manufacture its own corticosteroids, a substance which is required in the critical situation. (This can be counteracted with the administration of extra corticosteroids.)

Be prepared if you are one of those individuals who are prone to life-threatening reactions. If you don't own one, obtain an allergy kit for the house as well as for the car. Know how to use it and make sure your closest of kin know how too. Check the adrenaline every month for discoloration, which indicates deterioration, and make sure it is not out of date. Store it away from sunlight, which also causes adrenaline to deteriorate.

Post the name of your doctor near every telephone in your home. Consider wearing a medical information tag listing any and all the items to which you are allergic, or keep a card discloses this information on your person at all times.

Appendix B

A Handful of Simple Recipes

Here are a few "cook-less" easy to prepare extras for the time conscious that offer meal appeal.

Delightful Dressings

Tasty Vinegar and Oil Dressing

• Balsamic vinegar
• Olive oil
• Garlic powder

Mix 1 part vinegar and 1 part oil. Add a touch of garlic powder.

Balsamic vinegar supplies a subtle sweetness and the garlic powder gives the final product a little zest. This dressing is great in salads or to dip broccoli or other raw vegetables into.

Butter Dressing

• Olive oil
• Butter flavoring
• Sea salt

Add a drop or 2 of butter flavoring to several spoonfuls of oil. Pepper in sea salt.

This dressing is also fitting in salads or to dip raw vegetables into. It's excellent for those who are fond of butter, but must give it up.

"'Candy-less' Candy"

Date Nut Delight

• Medjool dates
• Pecans or Brazil nuts
• Wheat germ or cream of tartar

Pit dates. Replace seed with pecans or Brazil nuts. Roll in wheat germ or sprinkle on cream of tartar.

Obviously, if allergic to wheat, use cream of tartar. It will put in a little punch into the flavor. This holds psychological benefits as well, because the cream of tartar, by sight, resembles powdered sugar. It makes the final product attractive to the eye, still pleasing to the palate, and distracts one from taking in refined sweeteners.

Walnut-Raisin Goodie

• Raisins
• Walnuts
• Sesame seeds

Run ingredients through food chopper. Remove and form into balls. Roll in sesame seeds.

This sweet treat is excellent for those without sensitivity to nuts. It is both wheat-free and dairy-free and should satisfy any sweet tooth.

Frozen "Fruities"

Strawberry-Banana Nut Icy

- Bananas
- Strawberries
- Honey
- Almond slivers

Peel and slice bananas and remove strawberry leaves. Add one teaspoon of honey for every banana used. Run the fruits through blender. Pour into pint containers and top with almond slivers. Freeze, allow to thaw, then serve.

If strawberries are unavailable, add a few drops of strawberry flavoring. This is a good substitute for ice cream sundaes.

Apple Popsicles

- Apples
- Cinnamon

Run apples and a dash of cinnamon through blender. Pour into ice trays and add ice cream sticks to each block, then freeze.

This makes an excellent treat for the kids. If apple is not preferred, try another fruit. It is better to make your own fruit juice rather than depending on commercially processed drinks, which are less nourishing. If you desire strictly the juice, use a food processor. However, it you use a blender, it will give the final product more body—and it will be more nourishing, as the pulp of the fruit will be retained. The ice cubes can also be used to spice up drinks.

"Bodyful" Beverages

Pina Colada Shake

- Fresh pineapple
- Coconut flavoring

Chop pineapple and add to blender along with a few drops of coconut flavoring. Mix into a drink, pour, and serve immediately.

This is an excellent no-fat beverage which is nevertheless filling. It is better served fresh. Storing in the refrigerator for even one day will allow it to lose food value.

Peach Shake

- Peaches
- Nutmeg

Slice peaches and add to blender along with a dash of nutmeg. Mix into a drink and serve immediately.

This is another excellent no-fat, but equally filling drink. It too is better served fresh, as is any fruit or vegetable juice, because produce quickly loses food value after it is sliced.

Glossary

Allergen: An antigen that provokes an allergic reaction

Allergic rhinitis: The medical term for hay fever

Allergy: An adverse reaction in a person who has previously been exposed to a specific foreign substance and is exposed to it again.

Anaphylactic shock (anaphylaxis): A potentially fatal allergic reaction characterized by a rapid pulse, falling blood pressure, swollen throat, and fluid in the lungs

Antibodies: Proteins produced by the body that are tailor-made to match each specific substance in order to fight off infections and disease

Antigen: a foreign substance causing the production of an antibody when introduced into the human system, which may or may not induce an allergic reaction

Antihistamine: A medication that prevents symptoms such as congestion, runny nose, and sneezing by blocking or reducing the action of histamine

Dander: Tiny flakes of dead skin shed by people and animals

Decongestant: Any substance that relieves nasal congestion

Dust mites (dermatophagoides): Microscopic creatures found in dust that feed on flakes of skin and other food particles and are common triggers for allergies

Eczema: Inflammation of the skin that typically causes itching and sometimes accompanied by scaling, crusting, and oozing

Elimination diet: A diet in which certain foods are temporarily given up in order to rule them out as an allergen

Epinephrine: A form of adrenaline medication used for the purpose of treating anaphylactic shock and other severe allergic reactions

Glue ear (chronic secretory otitis media): A condition that results from an excessive accumulation of mucus in the nasal passages that works its way up into the eustachian tube to create an obstruction

Gluten: A protein found in wheat and other grains that can cause allergic reactions

Hay fever (allergic rhinitis): An allergic reaction characterized by acute inflammation of the eyes and upper respiratory tract

HEPA filter: A high-efficiency particulate air filter designed to remove a large percentage of particles from the air

Histamine: A naturally occurring substance released by the body following exposure to an allergen

Hypoallergenic: Products formulated to contain the least possible number of allergens and therefore less likely to trigger allergy

Keratin: A protein forming the principle matter of hair, nails, skin, etc.

Lactase: An enzyme in the body designed specifically to digest lactose

Lactose: The principle carbohydrate of milk

Outgassing: The gradual release of chemicals in plastics, rubber, synthetic fabrics, paints, glues, and the like due to curing or aging

Particulate matter: Matter composed of particles, as opposed to gaseous matter, or that which is made up of gas

Parvalbumins: Proteins contained in seafood that can trigger allergic reactions

Phenylethylamine: A substance contained in chocolate suspected of triggering allergic reactions

Photosensitivity: The state of being sensitive to sunlight, sometimes induced by certain medications

Pollinosis: Hay fever

Sebum: The oily substance that is secreted by the sebaceous glands

Sinusitis: Inflammation of the sinuses

Sulfonamides: A family of drugs designed to aid the body in overcoming infections, but sometimes responsible for allergic reactions

Bibliography

Berger, William E., Debra L. Gordon, Allergy & Asthma Relief. Pleasantville, New York: Reader's Digest Association.

Brody, Jane, Jane Brody's Allergy Fighter. New York, New York: W. W. Norton & Company, 1997.

Brostoff, Jonathan, M. D., Linda Gamlin. Hay Fever: The Complete Guide, Rochester, Vermont: Healing Arts Press, 2002.

Conry, Tom, Consumer's Guide to Cosmetics. Garden City, New York: Doubleday and Company, Inc., 1980.

Dadd, Debra Lynn, Nontoxic, Natural, & Earthwise. Los Angeles: Jeremy P. Tarcher, Inc., 1990.

Faelten, Sharon, Editors of Prevention Magazine. The Allergy Self-Help Book, Emmaus, Pennsylvania: Rodale Press, 1983.

Gabler, Raymond, Editors of Consumer Reports Books. Is Your Water Safe to Drink? Mount Vernon, New York: Consumer's Union, 1988.

Golos, Natalie, Frances Golos Golbitz, Coping with Your Allergies. New York, New York: Simon and Schuster, 1979.

Hunter, Beatrice Trum, Consumer Beware: Your Food and What's Been Done to It. New York, New York: Simon and Schuster, 1971.

Kattel, Mary S., The Doctor's Book of Home Remedies for Airborne Allergies. Rodale, 2000.

Melina, Vesanto, MS, RD, Jo Stepaniak, MSEd, Dina Aronson, MS, RD, Food Allergy Survival Guide. Summertown, Tennessee: Healthy Living Publications, 2004.

Rousseau, David, W. J. Rea, M. D., Jean Enwright, Your Home, Your Health, and Well-Being. Vancouver, B. C.: 1987.

Silverman, Harold M., The Pill Book: 10th Revised Edition. New York, New York: Bantam Books, 2002.

Steinman, David, Diet for a Poisoned Planet. New York, New York: Harmony Books, 1990.

Winter, Ruth, A Consumer's Dictionary of Food Additives. New York, New York: Crown Publishers, Inc., 1984.

Zamm, Alfred V., Why Your House May Endanger Your Health. New York, New York: Simon and Schuster, 1980.

Index of Tables

Index